Queer and Trans M

Merrick Daniel Pilling

Queer and Trans Madness

Struggles for Social Justice

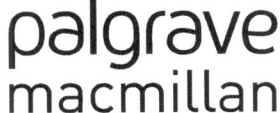

Merrick Daniel Pilling
Women's and Gender Studies
University of Windsor
Windsor, ON, Canada

ISBN 978-3-030-90415-9   ISBN 978-3-030-90413-5   (eBook)
https://doi.org/10.1007/978-3-030-90413-5

Cover image: Bad Air/Yer Grievances, 2018 © Christina Quarles. Courtesy of the artist, Hauser & Wirth, and Pilar Corrias, London

This Palgrave Macmillan imprint is published by the registered company Springer Nature Switzerland AG
The registered company address is: Gewerbestrasse 11, 6330 Cham, Switzerland

Acknowledgments

This book would not have been possible without the 37 people who participated as interviewees. I am profoundly grateful for their willingness to share their insights and experiences. I am thankful to Marc Stein, Geoffrey Reaume, and Sheila Cavanagh, who supported the Queer and Trans Madness project, one of the two studies on which this book is based. Many thanks to Andrea Daley for bringing me onto the second study on which this book is based, the Cultural Representations of Gender project, and providing feedback on Chapter 5. Thank you to Maria Khan for administrative support in preparing the manuscript. I am grateful for the helpful feedback provided by two anonymous peer reviewers. Many thanks to Christina Quarles for the use of Bad Air/Yer Grievances (2018) on the cover. Last but not least, I could not have finished this book without the love and support of my partner, Keith.

Financial support was received from the Ontario Graduate Scholarship Program and the Gender, Feminist, and Women's Studies Program at York University. Chapter 5 draws on research supported by the Social Sciences and Humanities Research Council.

Contents

1

Introduction: Queer and Trans Madness: Struggles for Social Justice

This book has been a long time in the making. Much has changed since I conceptualized the first of two research studies on which this book is based. I conducted the fieldwork in Winnipeg, Manitoba, and Toronto, Ontario, between 2010 and 2012, before the ideas and concepts that are foundational to Mad Studies had fully taken on that moniker.[1] They had long existed in the mad movement and in various bodies of scholarship, but the past 10 years have seen the establishment of Mad Studies as an academic field of study and an explosion of its growth in Canada and internationally, from the publication of the seminal text *Mad Matters: A Critical Reader in Canadian Mad Studies* in 2013 to the creation of a graduate program in Mad Studies at Queen Margaret University in Edinburgh, Scotland, in 2021.

My own introduction to what has become known as Mad Studies was in 2008, in Geoffrey Reaume's York University graduate course titled Mad People's History. This course introduced me to an inter-disciplinary body of work that provides "critique and transcendence of psy-centred ways of thinking, behaving, relating, and being" (LeFrançois et al., 2013, p. 13) and gives primacy to the voices of those with lived experience of mental distress, sidelining those usually considered the

© The Author(s), under exclusive license to Springer Nature Switzerland AG 2022
M. D. Pilling, *Queer and Trans Madness*,
https://doi.org/10.1007/978-3-030-90413-5_1

experts on these matters (Reaume, 2006). The ideologies that underpin Mad Studies helped me make sense of some my own life experiences, including the death of my cousin by suicide. I had long felt ill at ease with narrow constructions of distress and the impacts of trauma and structural oppression as individualized manifestations of mental illness. Mad Studies gave me the tools to reconceptualize many of the "personal, social, and ethical problems in living" that I had previously understood as being the result of chemical imbalance in the brain and genetic, medical conditions (Szasz, 1961, p. 262). This de-medicalizing of everyday life resonated with my longstanding resistance to the pathologizing of my queerness and transness. And yet, I found that the voices of queer and trans people, as well as those of Black, Indigenous, and people of colour (BIPOC), were not a strong presence in what I had seen of Mad Studies thus far.

This was part of my motivation for creating the first of two studies on which this book is based. As a doctoral candidate in Gender, Feminist and Women's Studies at York University, I was well versed in how white, cisnormative feminism had come to dominate the mainstream movement and some academic Women's Studies programs, leading to the exclusion and erasure of the histories, experiences, and contributions of feminists of colour and trans people (and the advent of trans-exclusionary radical feminists). I witnessed changes in the field that addressed these exclusions to varying degrees, and the eventual renaming of most Women's Studies programs (including my doctoral program) to variations on Women's and Gender Studies. As Mad Studies was taking shape, I wanted to contribute to this nascent field in a way that avoided replicating these same exclusions (Gorman et al., 2013). I conducted a qualitative study about the experiences of mad queer and trans people, for which I interviewed 37 lesbian, gay, bisexual, trans, and queer (LGBTQ)[2] people who had experienced mental distress, 15 of whom were BIPOC. In this study, I explored intersectional forms of oppression within the mental health system, workplaces (see Pilling, 2013), and mental health policy (see Pilling, 2019). It also allowed me to explore the fraught relationship between the concept of "mental illness" and LGBTQ people by applying a Mad Studies lens to explicate how the biomedical model is entrenched in, and perpetuates, cisnormative, heteronormative, white supremacist, and colonial ideologies.

Four years after I conducted the first study, I began the extraction of the data for the second study on which Chapter 5 of this book is based.[3] This project examined how psychiatry and the psychiatric institution are implicated in the organization of gender relations at the intersection of race, Indigeneity, sexuality, class, and disability. It investigated how psychiatric discourses participate in the (re)production and sanctioning of gendered ways of being distressed. By using psychiatric inpatient charts as texts for analysis, this study engaged in a process of "studying up" (Harding & Norberg, 2005) to reveal the power of institutional ideology (McColl et al., 2013; Moosa-Mitha, 2005) to reinscribe oppressive social and structural relations. I spent two years deeply engaged with 161 inpatient charts of people who were discharged from a large psychiatric institution in Ontario between 2013 and 2016.[4] I read and analysed thousands of pages of chart documentation written by psychiatrists, social workers, nurses, pharmacists, and recreational therapists.

In many ways, this experience changed my perspective and further convinced me of the need for Mad Studies and activism to illuminate and challenge the "psy complex" (LeFrançois et al., 2016). In particular, it deepened my understanding of the profundity of institutional violence and the power of institutional ideology to perpetuate and maintain structural white supremacy and colonialism, cisnormativity, and heteronormativity. Studying these charts showed me beyond a shadow of a doubt that BIPOC and trans, non-binary, and queer people[5] cannot safely rely on the mental health system as a means to address their mental distress. The charts also confirmed the narratives of the interviewees in the first study regarding structural oppression in the mental health system but in many ways elucidated the issues more starkly. The charts revealed the full force of psychiatric violence, including involuntary admissions (incarceration), forced drugging (often long-acting injectables), locked seclusion (solitary confinement), chemical and mechanical restraints applied forcibly with the aid of security guards, and electroconvulsive therapy (ECT). Some of the participants in the first study had been institutionalized and had experienced some of these things, but most had not, pointing to how their narratives were shaped by a certain level of privilege.

In 2019 I taught Mad People's History at X University's School of Disability Studies.[6] This version was based on a course originally created by David Reville and revised by Danielle Landry and Jenna Reid.[7] Teaching this course gave me the opportunity to reflect on the many developments in activist and scholarly work related to madness and Mad Studies that had transpired in the 11 years between taking Mad People's History at York University and teaching it at X University, for example, the establishment of the Black Lives Matter movement following the 2013 acquittal of George Zimmerman in the murder of Trayvon Martin, and relatedly, the theorizing of anti-Black sanism (Abdillahi et al., 2017; Meerai et al., 2016), misogynoir, and transmisogynoir (Bailey & Trudy, 2018). There was also the further growth of Disability Justice as a movement and framework rooted in the knowledge of mad and disabled queer and trans, BIPOC (Bernes, 2015; Piepzna-Samarasinha, 2018). Exclusions in the field persist, most notably that Mad Studies has mainly been a project of the Global North, with some exceptions (Davar, 2015; Mills & Fernando, 2014; Mills, 2014, 2017; MindFreedom Ghana, 2019; Nabbali, 2013).[8] The forthcoming volume *The Routledge International Handbook of Mad Studies* may begin to address this gap (Beresford & Russo, 2022). As I wrote part of this book, a global pandemic and a global uprising against anti-Black racism following the murder of George Floyd in 2020 by police rocked the world and raised mainstream (whitestream) awareness of systemic anti-Black racism, as well as concepts such as mutual aid and collective care. All of these activist and scholarly interventions have aided my own (un)learning as well as contributed to my flagging faith in the state and institutions since conceptualizing and undertaking the first study that informs this book.

Much has changed since I conducted the interviews for the first study, and yet, in many ways, the participants' narratives read as if the interviews took place yesterday. A study I worked on from 2018 to 2020 further confirmed for me that many of the issues identified in both studies persist, illuminating the tenacity of these problems from yet another angle. For this most recent project, I co-created and delivered workshops to service providers regarding trauma-informed care for two-spirit, lesbian, gay, bisexual, trans, and queer (2SLGBTQ) people.[9] I travelled across Ontario to deliver these workshops and met all manner of kind and passionate practitioners working in mental health, social services, and anti-violence initiatives. Over and over again, I heard that the information provided in the training was something these practitioners had not encountered previously, especially when it came to working with trans and non-binary people. This demonstrates enduring structural deficits in education and the persistence of transphobia, cisnormativity, racism, and other forms of oppression that lead to service providers being gravely ill-equipped to serve trans and queer people, especially BIPOC, despite their best intentions.

There have been studies conducted since the completion of my first study that demonstrate that queer and trans people continue to face oppression in mental health services. However, there has yet to be a comprehensive application of Mad Studies to queer and trans experiences of mental distress despite the natural fit of, and overlap between, the two. The primary aim of this book is to do just that. There is certainly mental health research concerning LGBTQ people, and the past decade has seen growth in scholarship in this area. However, as I will explain, this research is distinct from Mad Studies in several ways.

Mental health research often positions LGBTQ people as an at-risk or vulnerable group concerning mental health because of the widespread nature of homophobia, transphobia, and other forms of oppression. According to this body of work, there is a higher prevalence of mental health problems among LGBTQ people, in part because of experiences of societal discrimination based on sexuality, gender identity, race, and class (Chamberland & Saewyc, 2012; Khan et al., 2017; Ross, Gibson, et al., 2018; Ross, Salway, et al., 2018; Rotondi, Bauer, Scanlon, et al. 2012; Rotondi, Bauer, Travers, et al., 2011; Sutter & Perrin, 2016; Williams et al., 2017). Within this body of work, some scholars employ the minority-stress model, in which stress brought on by homophobia and transphobia are seen as triggers of mental illness or mental health problems (Brooks, 1981; Hatzenbuehler, 2009; Meyer, 2003; Morrison, 2011).

Some of these studies also document the failings of the mental health system to provide easily accessible, affirming care for LGBTQ people, arguing that in some cases this results in unmet mental health needs and untreated illness (McIntyre et al., 2011; Simeonov et al., 2015; Steele et al., 2017; Williams et al., 2017). Many also include recommendations for improving access to, and the quality of, mental health care services for LGBTQ people to better suit their needs (Robertson et al., 2015; Ross, Gibson, et al., 2018). Many of these studies are conducted by LGBTQ-identified and allied researchers, whose aims are to provide empirical proof of the negative health impacts of homophobia and transphobia in order to bolster the legitimacy and necessity of eradicating such oppression across various contexts and improving LGBTQ mental health.

This scholarship is distinct from Mad Studies, which challenges the overarching ideology that mental distress is a disease. For example, claims that LGBTQ people are more 'vulnerable' to mental disorders or have a higher prevalence of 'mental health problems' do not challenge the concept of mental illness and the medicalization of distress even while they acknowledge the role of social factors in contributing to distress. To be clear, the studies described above are not monolithic in the extent to which they endorse an illness model of distress. For example, a minority acknowledge (but do not fully explore) the limitations of the biomedical model, such as the ways in which it individualizes systemic oppression (McIntyre et al., 2011; Ross, Gibson, et al., 2018). Scholars who employ the minority stress model are especially prone to positioning social factors (such as homophobia and transphobia) as secondary to biological considerations. As Johnstone (2011) notes about similar vulnerability-stress models, such theories give primacy to "the 'biological' and by so doing reduce[s] other factors ('stresses') to the lesser status of 'triggers' of the underlying 'illness', thus divesting them of their personal meaning and preserving biomedical assumptions relatively intact" (p. 102). As Boyle (2011) also notes, the vulnerability-stress model (and others like it) undermine the importance of adverse life experiences by implying that "negative experiences are not inherently stressful but are made so by pre-existing vulnerability so that only 'the vulnerable' are adversely affected – 'normal' people would be able to cope" (pp. 31–32). The portrayal of exploited groups as 'vulnerable' also places the focus on 'disordered' individuals rather than the exploitative systems that create marginalization. Mainstream mental health research on LGBTQ people is thus distinct from Mad Studies because to varying degrees, it upholds a biomedical model, even while providing important analyses of the role of oppression in causing distress. Further, calls for inclusive and LGBTQ-affirming care, while important, are different from a Mad Studies approach, which might document and critique the harms of psychiatrization and the violence inflicted by, and entrenched in, psychiatric knowledge production and the mental health system itself (rather than solely in society at large).

Much of mainstream mental research on LGBTQ people can also be seen as an example of what Tuck (2009), writing in the context of research conducted about Indigenous peoples, calls "damage-centred research" (p. 409). Tuck defines damage-centered research as that which "operates, even benevolently, from a theory of change that establishes harm or injury in order to achieve reparation" (p. 413). Damage-centred research positions "entire communities as depleted" (p. 409) and is more insidious than blatantly "damaging research" because it takes social context and oppression into account:

> In damaged-centered research, one of the major activities is to document pain or loss in an individual, community, or tribe. Though connected to deficit models—frameworks that emphasize what a particular student, family, or community is lacking to explain underachievement or failure—damage-centered research is distinct in being more socially and historically situated. It looks to historical exploitation, domination, and colonization to explain contemporary brokenness, such as poverty, poor health, and low literacy. Common sense tells us this is a good thing, but the danger in damage-centred research is that it is a pathologizing approach in which the oppression singularly defines a community. (p. 413)

Damage-centred mental health research can be aligned with popular discourses that position LGBTQ communities as undesirable and irrevocably broken, although it is very different in its underlying intent.

This is perhaps a controversial claim, because it stands in contrast to the general consensus of contemporary mainstream mental health research on LGBTQ people; it is seen as progressive because it moves away from previous understandings of LGBTQ people as inherently disordered because of gender and sexual nonconformity. Those invested in social justice for 2SLGBTQ people generally understand that the explicit pathologizing of 2SLGBTQ people through specific diagnoses in the *Diagnostic and Statistical Manual of Mental Disorders* (DSM) is problematic and contentious.[10] However, a broad critique of the biomedical model like the one I employ in this book is not widely embraced, including within 2SLGBTQ communities.

In some ways, the process of declassifying homosexuality as a mental disorder in the DSM in the 1970s exposed the enculturated character of psychiatry as a whole, revealing the ways in which psychiatric designations of "normal" and "abnormal" were intricately tied to predominant social values (Bayer, 1987). However, as discussed in Chapter 2, the larger emancipatory implications of this blow to the foundations of psychiatry and mainstream mental health practice have not been realized. Those invested in social justice for 2SLGBTQ people have focused on the depathologizing of specific diagnoses pertaining to sexuality and gender identity rather than challenging the broad medicalization of distress and its impact on LGBTQ people. This narrow focus on the pathologizing of specific diagnoses leads to the mistaken belief that once such diagnoses are removed from the DSM, gender and sexual dissidence (and 2SLGBTQ people) will no longer be pathologized. I argue otherwise in this book and employ a Mad Studies lens to demonstrate that pathologizing distress is not necessarily better than pathologizing identity.

Mad Studies offers an alternative to the damage-centred mainstream mental health research on LGBTQ people, though, in some ways, my arguments are similar to this literature. For example, I support the contention that oppression of all kinds, including homophobia, transphobia, sanism, ableism, sexism, classism, and racism have negative effects on 2SLGBTQ people. Indeed, I argue throughout this book that oppression can contribute or lead to mental distress. However, this is not the same as the claim made in much of the mainstream LGBTQ mental health research that LGBTQ people are more 'vulnerable' to mental disorders or mental health problems. As noted, the latter is limited in that it does not challenge the concept of mental illness and the medicalization of distress. One of the aims of this book is to show that Mad Studies facilitates a broad critique of the biomedical model and that this lens is more aligned with achieving social justice for 2SLGBTQ people than an individualizing biomedical model, or damage-centred mental health research (Tuck, 2009).

Employing a Mad Studies lens, I question the need to medicalize experiences and behaviours that are labeled mental illness and mental health problems, not because mental illness is undesirable, but because the biomedical model is steeped in oppressive ideologies about 2SLGBTQ people and BIPOC and reduces the effects of violence and trauma to individual deficits while also sometimes perpetuating harm and violence through treatment. While respecting that some 2SLGBTQ people and BIPOC choose to use medical strategies to address their mental distress, I question their efficacy, especially given the vexed context in which this occurs for 2SLGBTQ people and BIPOC. I argue that further incorporating queer and trans people into mental health systems can run counter to the desired goal of improving health and may, in fact, result in iatrogenic harm and punitive approaches to treatment and recovery that elide autonomy.

I argue that change both within and outside of the mental healthcare system is necessary. There are many 2SLGBTQ people who want to, or are forced to, use mental health services. Based on a critical analysis of participant narratives and chart documentation, this book discusses changes within the mental healthcare system and social services more broadly that would make them more liveable for 2SLGBTQ people. In this way, I make some claims that are reminiscent of the damage-centred mainstream research on LGBTQ mental health. However, I also explore the ways in which mad 2SLGBTQ people can, and already do, create non-carceral, non-state interventionist responses to mental distress, while recognizing that there is significant oppression within our communities, necessitating ongoing anti-sanist, anti-ableist, anti-racist, and decolonizing work.

My overarching goal in writing this book is to urge those interested in social justice for 2SLGBTQ people to consider the benefits of broadening the critique beyond the depathologization of specific diagnoses and to be cautious about advocating for more access to treatment without critically examining what constitutes treatment and the impact of medicalized strategies, including carceral and coercive tactics, on mad 2SLGBTQ people. A mad-queer-trans lens is essential because it is grounded within a broad critique of the biomedical model while looking specifically at how gender and sexual dissidence, and therefore 2SLGBTQ people, are psychiatrized and how these dynamics are also racialized. A mad-queer-trans lens supports queer and trans bodily autonomy and counters anti-queer and anti-trans practices of all kinds. My hope is to further realize the emancipatory promise of queer and trans madness, which I see as making more space to exist as mad, queer and trans, with more resources to respond to crisis and distress in ways that are non-coercive and non-carceral, and honour autonomy as well as interdependence within our communities.

Language: Sexuality and Gender Identity

Language is dynamic, shifting and changing over time according to the needs of its users. In a heteronormative, cisnormative world, language creation is one of the ways that those who live outside the norms of sexuality and gender resist normative frameworks and imposed labels, and build community with one another. Terminology is critically important in self-determination as well as in collective, community understandings of identities, experiences, and ways of being that have been violently suppressed and marginalized. It is, therefore, important to carefully consider and explain my use of language and terminology.

Throughout this book, I employ "queer" and "trans" as umbrella terms that encompass a longer list of identities such as lesbian, gay, bisexual, transgender, and genderqueer. However, I also use the acronym "LGBTQ" to refer to the participants from the first study (henceforth referred to as "the participants"). While many (62%) used the term queer as at least one of their self-designations, there were enough who did not to warrant the use of LGBTQ in addition to queer and trans, in order not to completely subsume those who used other terms. It is important to note that LGBTQ still subsumes and excludes some identities. As noted, I aim to be deliberate in the use of the acronym LGBTQ, which stands for lesbian, gay, bisexual, trans, and queer and the use of the acronym 2SLGBTQ, which stands for two spirit, lesbian, gay, bisexual, trans, and queer. I use the acronym LGBTQ when referring to the interview participants in study one because none of the six participants who self-identified as Métis or Indigenous identified as two-spirit.[11] Chapters 3 and 4, which focus on the results of study one, employ the acronym LGBTQ instead of 2SLGBTQ for this reason. Throughout the book I also use the acronym LGBTQ when referring to bodies of research, activist organizing, and community spaces, that exclude two-spirit people. In most other instances I use the acronym 2SLGBTQ, including when referring to some of the broader implications of my research.

Notably, the "T" that stands for "trans" still serves as an umbrella term for trans, transgender, and genderqueer. At the time of interviewing in 2010–2012, the term "genderqueer" was in frequent use, whereas the term "non-binary" was not. It was also more common than it is today to identify both as a woman or a man and as genderqueer. With the rise of the term non-binary, it has become increasingly customary not to subsume genderqueer and non-binary under the umbrella of trans. However, this was not the case at the time of interviewing. In Chapter 5, which focuses on the chart documentation data from study two, I use the phrase "trans and non-binary" because it reflects the specific demographics of the people included in that study.

As noted, I employ queer as an umbrella term and an identity category, but I also make use of the term queer as a concept. Early uses of queer in the late 1980s and 90s by academics and activists such as Queer Nation were often anti-identitarian. Queer was seen as impossible to fully define, "a zone of possibilities" (Edelman, 1994, p. 114). Queer shifted the focus from identity to acts, desires, bodies, and performances, drawing attention to "mismatches between sex, gender and desire" (Jagose, 1996, p. 3). The concept of queer also signalled resistance to homonormative, cisnormative identities, experiences, and ways of being in the world. When I make use of the term queer throughout this book, it is sometimes in this sense, despite the increasing political neutralizing of the term in recent years.

Language: The Biomedical Model of Mental Illness

Throughout this book, I employ the phrase "the biomedical model of mental illness" (or "the biomedical model," or "biomedicalism"). Use of this language sometimes leads to concerns about overgeneralization. I understand this concern to be based in the desire to differentiate between the various approaches and perspectives encompassed within the psy complex. There certainly are vast differences between psychiatry and psychology, for example, not to mention the many different approaches within each discipline, including some that consider social context (such as the biopsychosocial model of psychiatry and community psychology). There are other important distinctions, such as that only psychiatrists and other medical doctors have the power to prescribe medication and drug people against their will, though other types of practitioners (including psychologists, social workers, psychotherapists, and others) can, and do, convince people of the merit of taking medications or voluntarily presenting to medical/psychiatric facilities.

However, I use the language of biomedical model instead of something more narrow like biopsychiatry to draw attention to the common assumptions that underpin the vast majority of mental health service provisions including psychiatry, psychology, and social work, but extending far beyond formal medical settings into public policy, popular culture, and everyday language. The ideology that unites them despite their vast differences categorizes various experiences, behaviours, and thought patterns as indicative of biological deficiencies that can be scientifically evidenced and universally applied. Lewis (2006) describes the main tenets of biomedicalism as follows: mental illness is a disabling, biological deficiency that is "accompanied by physical pathology" and can be "classified as distinct disorders that have characteristic common features" (p. 107). Further, the causes of mental illness can be explained "in terms of physical illness" such as brain structure, genetics, and biochemistry (p. 107). The biomedical model of mental illness is currently predominant, so much so that in a tautological form of reasoning, the refusal to accept the biomedical model as a way of making sense of one's own experiences is seen as evidence of mental illness (Pilling et al., 2018; Ringer & Holen, 2016). Rimke (2016), in her theorizing of psychocentrism, has usefully articulated the ideas underpinning biomedicalism as a form of oppression, which she defines as the "view that human problems are due to a biologically-based flaw or deficit in the bodies and/or minds of individual subjects. Psychocentrism is itself a form of social injustice, where individual reformation rather than social and economic justice is promoted" (p. 5). At times, I employ the term psychocentrism as well.

While psychiatry as a medical science is most obviously informed by biomedicalism, this perspective also extends to psychology and beyond. As Rapley et al. (2011) state, "mainstream psychology…while sometimes appearing to offer alternative approaches, essentially supports the positivist psychiatric project of codifying human suffering into disease-like categories" (p. 1). There are versions of psychiatry and psychology that place more emphasis on social context, but as Beresford (2005) claims, even these "have taken as given the over-arching medicalised framework of 'mental illness,' although differing in the extent to which they saw it as a consequence of nature or nurture" (p. 36). The same claim has been made about social work practice and education (Poole et al., 2012). Seemingly ubiquitous, the biomedical view of mental illness extends well beyond formal medical contexts. It is evident in anti-stigma campaigns that compare mental illness to a disease like any other, in news stories that attribute violent behaviour to mentally ill perpetrators, and in television shows like *Cracked* (2013) and *Ratched* (2020) and blockbuster movies such as *A Beautiful Mind* (2001) and *Black Swan* (2010). Therefore, when I refer to the biomedical model of mental illness, I am invoking a concept much larger than that which forms the basis of the medical practice of psychiatry.

Further, as a text situated within Mad Studies, this book does not attempt to present a 'balanced' view of biomedicalism and the mental health system and, in fact, denies that there is such a thing as a balanced view. No position or analysis is politically neutral; it is just more likely to be labeled as political or ideological when the argument challenges the status quo and what is commonly accepted as truth. At a time when the biomedical model is firmly entrenched in health care, academic scholarship, public policy, and mainstream discourse, robust critiques are both outnumbered and necessary.

Language: Madness and Mental Health

As indicated by its name, Mad Studies rejects the language of biomedicalism and makes use of alternative language and terminology. Throughout this book I employ two such terms: "mental distress" and "madness." Tew (2011) contends that "perhaps more than in any other field of health and social care, language relating to mental health issues is contested and contentious" (p. 4). Choices regarding language and naming are critically important not only because they are indicative of an ideological stance, but because of the violence that can be enacted through labelling. As Price (2011) argues, "the problem of naming…acquires a particular urgency when considered in the context of disabilities of the mind, for often the very terms used to name persons with mental disabilities have explicitly foreclosed our status *as* persons" (p. 9; emphasis original).

Some activists and scholars who critique the biomedical model suggest that we refuse to use medical language such as mental illness (Boyle, 2011; Burstow, 2013; Tew, 2011). Burstow (2013) contends that when this language is used, "we are performing our designated role in the work of psychiatry…we are activating it" (p. 82). "Mental distress" has been proposed as an alternative because, unlike the term mental illness, it does not "do violence to people's identities and aspirations" and it "does not imply illness, incapacity, or inferiority" (Tew, 2011, p. 5). Likewise, "madness" has been politicized by those who resist the medicalization of distress with the goal of "reclaiming disparaged identities and restoring dignity and pride to difference" (LeFrançois et al., 2013, p. 10). Madness also captures a "broad historical sweep" and acknowledges that biomedicalism is just one of many ways in which such matters have been understood (Price, 2011, p. 10).

In addition to referring to madness and mental distress, I also make use of the phrase "mental health," as it has been institutionalized as an umbrella term to describe mental well-being, various states of mind, and what are often understood as mental health 'disorders' (for example, by the Canadian Mental Health Association and the Mental Health Commission of Canada). When the participants in my study and I were talking, we often used the phrase "mental health" because this language structured their everyday lives, especially in health care settings but also at work and in everyday practices. I, therefore, also use this term as an acknowledgement of the current context in which madness is understood and thus the ways in which the research participants were positioned. Mental health was the predominant framework available to them to make sense of themselves. However, I make use of this term carefully and selectively. As other scholars have argued, mental health is no less complicit with biomedical ideology than the term mental illness (Boyle, 2011; Burstow, 2013).

In referring to specific participants, I use pseudonyms. When referring to the participants as a group, I use the term mad and variations on the phrase "those who have experienced mental distress." As Diamond (2013) notes, the term mad can be used as an umbrella term to "describe people who have been labelled and treated as crazy" (p. 66). However, as will be explored in detail in Chapter 3, interviewees used a large variety of terms to refer to their identities including various psychiatric diagnoses, crazy, mad, psychiatric service user, psychiatric survivor, consumer, and mentally ill. This assortment of terms reflects the participants' range of approaches to conceptualizing madness or mental health. Some participants rejected the medical model of mental illness and eschewed medical labels altogether, choosing more politicized terms to describe themselves. Some used medical model language strategically, for example, to make themselves intelligible in certain contexts such as in healthcare facilities and their workplace. Others embraced the medical model and employed the term mentally ill unequivocally.

In Chapter 5, I make use of the term "patients" to describe the people to whom the charts belonged. I use this term because all of the individuals whose charts are included in the second study were psychiatric inpatients, some of them admitted involuntarily (incarcerated), and thus terms that imply more agency (e.g., survivor, client) are not applicable. Given the lack of information on self-identification and the context of the psychiatric institution, it seemed most appropriate to use the language of patient, which best reflects the unequal power relationships inherent in chart documentation. In short, I employ the term to indicate how they were interpellated by the psychiatric institution. In referring to specific chart records, however, I employ pseudonyms to facilitate discussion of the findings and to humanize the people to whom these charts belong.[12]

Mental Distress Is Real

I have found in sharing my work that critiques of the psy complex can be perceived as attacks on the veracity of firsthand experiences of distress. Those with experiential connections to concepts of mental illness may have strong personal investments in the truth of the biomedical model. This can invoke anger and "downright hostility" to the concept of madness and critiques of the biomedical model (LeFrançois et al., 2013, p. 11). Further, those who have been helped by medical strategies for addressing mental distress or who know those who have can feel as if those experiences are being invalidated, dismissed, or erased. It is important to be clear that mental distress is real and has material effects on the lives of those who experience it. It is also important to acknowledge that some find medical strategies, including psychiatric treatment and medications, helpful. For some people, including some participants in the first study, psychiatric medications and health professionals operating within a biomedical framework had been helpful and had made life more liveable. However, as discussed in Chapter 4, the participants also recounted experiences that indicated systemic racism, homophobia, transphobia, and other forms of oppression within the mental health system. Chapter 5 illustrates this more starkly through analyses of chart documentation written by mental health practitioners on inpatient units in a psychiatric hospital. The existence of good experiences within the system does not negate the prevalence of structural oppression, in the same way that illuminating the existence of structural oppression does not negate that good experiences can be had by some, often those with privilege in some respect(s) (on this last point see, also, Pilling et al. [2018]).

It bears repeating that I believe in self-identification and definition in whatever way feels right (including as mentally ill) and that everyone should be able to choose how they want to address their own experiences of mental distress (including medical strategies such as psychiatric drugs and admission to a psychiatric hospital). I also believe that true choice involves being able to choose *not to* use medical strategies. This is not currently the case; it is possible to be held involuntarily in a psychiatric facility; it is also possible to be deemed incapable of making treatment decisions, which can result in forced drugging or ECT. The choice not to rely on medical strategies also requires the existence of substantial alternatives, including support for withdrawing from psychiatric drugs, information about long-term outcomes based on research that is conducted independently of pharmaceutical companies, and demedicalized, non-carceral approaches to crisis response. Currently, the existence of such alternatives is limited, as I explore further in Chapter 6.

Organization of the Book

This book draws on data from two research studies.[13] Chapters 3, 4, and 6 draw on a subset of the data from the Queer and Trans Madness study (study one) focusing on interview data from 37 participants about mental distress, identity, community, and experiences in healthcare settings. Chapter 5 draws on a subset of the data from the Cultural Representations of Gender project (study two), focusing on 16 charts of trans and non-binary people.

Chapter 2 explores historical and contemporary tensions and overlaps in activist and scholarly interventions at the intersections of madness, queerness, and transness. I explore the origins of a single-issue politic in

LGBTQ activism that employed sanist logics in the service of declassifying homosexuality as a mental illness in the DSM as well as the existence of an intersectional, coalitional politic that was present at the time of declassification struggles. I discuss the scholarly outgrowths of these activist interventions and the possibilities of emerging scholarship using a mad-queer-trans lens. I suggest that ideas and activism that are often disparaged as belonging to the "lunatic fringe" are sources of subjugated knowledge that shed light on the mutually constitutive character of madness, queerness, and transness as well as intersectional analyses of structural racism, colonialism, sanism, homophobia, transphobia, classism, and other forms of oppression in the biomedical model of mental illness.

Drawing on data from study one, Chapter 3 advances a broad critique of the biomedical model while paying attention to the ways in which it specifically affects LGBTQ people. This chapter draws on 37 interviews with LGBTQ people who experienced mental distress, discussing their identification with various terms, identities, and diagnostic categories. However, it is not only a discussion of the different ways in which participants self-identified. The participants' rationales for rejecting or embracing various terminologies often pointed to fundamental problems with the biomedical model itself and indicated the value of a mad-queer-trans analytic.[14] While the biomedical model has become so predominant that it is difficult to conceptualize experiences of mental distress through any other lens, the participants' narratives clearly demonstrate some of the problems with biomedicalism and point to the benefits of applying insights from Mad Studies that take social context into account. I argue that a mad-queer-trans lens broadly challenges the biomedical model, indicating why it is crucial to expand the fight for depathologization of gender and sexual dissidence beyond a narrow focus on specific diagnoses concerning gender and sexual dissidence.

In many ways, Chapters 4 and 5 are companion chapters. While Chapter 4 details encounters between participants and mental health care practitioners from the perspective of the participants in study one, Chapter 5 analyses patient-practitioner encounters using practitioners' chart documentation from study two. Chapter 4 shows that the power relations embedded in biomedical practice create inequitable relationships between service providers and participants. Participant narratives show that structural heteronormativity, cisnormativity, racism, colonialism, and other forms of oppression in the mental health care system persist. This chapter challenges the notion that mental health care practitioners informed by biomedicalism perform objective assessments of participants' mental health and points to the problems with advocating for more access to mental health care without questioning the nature of what constitutes treatment.

Chapter 5 builds on the argument established in Chapter 4 regarding the subjective and discriminatory character of biomedical practice by examining chart documentation from study two regarding 16 trans and non-binary patients on inpatient units in a psychiatric hospital in Ontario. An analysis of these charts shows that cisnormativity governs the way trans people are treated in psychiatric settings and disrupts the idea that changing or removing gender identity-related diagnoses from the DSM will stop the pathologization of trans and non-binary people. This chapter demonstrates that psychiatric institutions can be unsafe places for trans and non-binary people, particularly those who are BIPOC. It also further demonstrates that advocating for more access to mental health treatment will not serve emancipatory aims when treatment continues to reinforce cisnormative, damaging assumptions about mental distress and gender dissidence.

The final chapter argues that change both within and outside of the mental health care system is necessary. Based on the analysis of participant narratives and chart documentation presented in Chapters 4 and 5 respectively, in the concluding chapter, I discuss the necessary change within the mental healthcare system to make it more liveable for 2SLGBTQ people who want to, or who are forced to, use it. Drawing on participant narratives from study one about mutual aid and collective care within queer and trans communities, this chapter also explores the ways mad 2SLGBTQ people create effective community responses to distress. I discuss some of the problems with carceral and state-interventionist responses to acute distress and suicidality and describe recent initiatives that offer other ways to respond. The book ends with a call to those invested in social justice for 2SLGBTQ people to interrogate the biomedical model of mental illness beyond the depathologization of gender and sexual dissidence and to further explore the emancipatory promise of queer and trans madness.

Acknowledgements Sections of this chapter draw on an earlier publication by the author: Daley, A., & Pilling, M. D. (2021). Introduction: Psychiatric documentation, power, and violence. In A. Daley & M. D. Pilling (Eds.), *Interrogating psychiatric narratives of madness: Documented lives* (pp. 1–32). Palgrave Macmillan.

Notes

1. Richard Ingram (2016) is credited with coining the term Mad Studies in 2008, though he describes this as a collective process: "I feel it was as if many people were playing a game of pass the parcel at a birthday party, and I happened to be the person who unwrapped the last layer of wrapping paper. Frankly, it could have been anyone in the circle who found themselves holding the newborn concept when the music stopped" (p. 12).
2. I aim to be deliberate in the use of the acronym LGBTQ, which stands for lesbian, gay, bisexual, trans, and queer and the use of the acronym 2SLGBTQ, which stands for two spirit, lesbian, gay, bisexual, trans, and queer. I use the acronym LGBTQ when referring to the interview participants in study one because none of the six research participants who were Indigenous or Métis identified as two-spirit. Chapters 3 and 4, which focus on the results of study one, employ the acronym LGBTQ instead of 2SLGBTQ for this reason. I also employ the acronym LGBTQ when referring to bodies of research, activist organizing, and community spaces, that exclude two-spirit people. In most other instances I use the acronym 2SLGBTQ, including when referring to some of the broader implications of my research.
3. Principle investigator on this project was Andrea Daley, and team members were Margaret Gibson, Lori Ross, Juveria Zaheer, and myself. It was shaped by input from community members Dawnmarie Harriott and Opal Sparks and completed with administrative assistance from Madeline Samsa. I worked on this study from May 2015 to January 2018.

4. I draw on a subset of this larger data set in Chapter Five, focusing on the 16 charts of trans and non-binary people. For analyses of the full data set see Daley and Pilling (2021) and Pilling et al. (2018).

5. These groups are obviously not mutually exclusive, but throughout this book I sometimes name BIPOC explicitly because of white supremacy. It is often the case that when BIPOC are not explicitly named, it is because their experiences have been erased.

6. For an explanation of the use of X University, see the open letter from Indigenous students at this university: https://yellowheadinstitute.org/2021/05/11/welcome-to-x-university-an-open-letter-to-the-community-from-indigenous-students/?fbclid=IwAR3IY4Qmb4mjU0G4Tau17bD5w uL3TQry41X8Y1Brzf5PcchJc2bYNCqoDrk.

7. For a discussion of this course and Mad Studies pedagogy, see Snyder et al. (2019).

8. I acknowledge that my own analyses are limited in this respect and are contextually specific to Canada, though I believe they are relevant to the Global North more broadly.

9. The principle investigator on this project was Lori Ross, and team members were Wesley Gos, Jenna MacKay, Michelle Tam, Olivia Taylor, and myself. The project was developed with the guidance of an Indigenous elder, Blu Waters, and a community advisory committee. See www.buildi ngcompetence.ca and www.lgbtqhealth.ca for more information.

10. There are significant differences between declassification struggles concerning homosexuality and trans-related diagnoses such as gender identity disorder and gender dsyphoria because such diagnoses greatly influence access to the technologies of medical transition for trans people.

11. For a discussion of the meaning of two-spirit, see Laing (2021).

12. For continuity, I use the same pseudonyms employed in my chapter and those by other research team members in the edited collection that presents analyses of the larger data set of 161 (see Daley & Pilling, 2021). It is, therefore, possible to easily identify analyses of the charts that were analysed in both volumes.

13. A discussion of the methodology for both studies can be found in the appendix. For further discussion of the methodology for the Cultural Representations of Gender study (study two) (see Daley & Pilling, 2021).

14. By "mad-queer-trans" I mean at the intersections of madness, queerness, and transness, and the order of these words is not important.

References

Abdillahi, I., Meerai, S., & Poole, J. (2017). When the suffering is compounded: Towards anti-Black sanism. In S. Wehbi & H. Parada (Eds.), *Reimagining anti-oppression social work practice* (pp. 109–122). Canadian Scholars Press.

Bailey, M., & Trudy. (2018). On misogynoir: Citation, erasure, and plagiarism. *Feminist Media Studies, 18*(4), 762–768. https://doi.org/10.1080/146 80777.2018.1447395

Bayer, R. (1987). *Homosexuality and American psychiatry*. Princeton University Press.

Beresford, P. (2005). Social approaches to madness and distress: User perspectives and user knowledges. In J. Tew (Ed.), *Social perspectives in mental health: Developing social models to understand and work with mental distress* (pp. 32–52). Jessica Kingsley Publishers.

Beresford, P., & Russo, J. (2022). *The Routledge international handbook of Mad Studies*. Routledge.

Bernes, P. (2015). *Disability justice—A working draft by Patty Berne*. Retrieved June 17, 2021, from https://www.sinsinvalid.org/blog/disability-justice-a-working-draft-by-patty-berne

Boyle, M. (2011). Making the world go away, and how psychology and psychiatry benefit. In M. Rapley, J. Moncrieff, & J. Dillon (Eds.), *De-medicalizing misery: Psychiatry, psychology and the human condition* (pp. 27–44). Palgrave Macmillan. https://doi.org/10.1057/9780230342507

Brooks, V. R. (1981). *Minority stress and lesbian women*. Lexington Books.

Burstow, B. (2013). A rose by any other name: Naming and the battle against psychiatry. In B. LeFrançois, R. Menzies, & G. Reaume (Eds.), *Mad matters: A critical reader in Canadian Mad Studies* (pp. 79–90). Canadian Scholars Press.

Chamberland, L., & Saewyc, E. (2012). Stigma, vulnerability, and resilience: The psychosocial health of sexual minority and gender diverse people in Canada. *Canadian Journal of Community Mental Health, 30*(2), 1–5. https://doi.org/10.7870/cjcmh-2011-0012

Daley, A., & Pilling, M. D. (2021). *Interrogating psychiatric narratives of madness: Documented lives*. Palgrave Macmillan.

Davar, B. V. (2015). Disabilities, colonization and globalisation: How the very possibility of a disability identity was compromised for the "insane" in India. In H. Spandler, J. Anderson, & B. Sapey (Eds.), *Madness, distress and the politics of disablement* (pp. 215–227). Policy Press. https://doi.org/10.1332/policypress/9781447314578.003.0016

Diamond, S. (2013). What makes us a community? Reflections on building solidarity in anti-sanist praxis. In B. A. LeFrançois, R. Menzies, & G. Reaume (Eds.), *Mad matters: A critical reader in Canadian Mad Studies* (pp. 64–78). Canadian Scholars Press.

Edelman, L. (1994). Homographesis: Essays in gay literary and cultural theory. *Routledge.* https://doi.org/10.4324/9781315889214

Gorman, R., saini, a., Tam, L., Udegbe, O., & Usar, O. (2013). Mad people of color—A manifesto. *Asylum,* 20(4), 27. Retrieved August 25, 2021, from https://asylummagazine.org/2013/12/mad-people-of-color-a-manifesto-by-rachel-gorman-annu-saini-louise-tam-onyinyechukwu-udegbe-onar-usar/

Harding, S., & Norberg, K. (2005). New feminist approaches to social science methodologies: An introduction. *Signs, 30*(4), 2009–2015. https://doi.org/10.1086/428420

Hatzenbuehler, M. (2009). How does sexual minority stigma get "under the skin"? A psychological mediation framework. *Psychological Bulletin, 135*(5), 707–730. https://doi.org/10.1037/a0016441

Ingram, R. A. (2016). Doing mad studies: Making (non)sense together. *Intersectionalities: A Global Journal of Social Work Analysis, Research, Polity, and Practice, 5*(3), 11–17. https://journals.library.mun.ca/ojs/index.php/IJ/article/view/1680/1327

Jagose, A. (1996). *Queer theory: An introduction.* New York University Press.

Johnstone, L. (2011). Can traumatic events traumatize people? Trauma, madness and "psychosis." In M. Rapley, J. Moncrieff, & J. Dillon (Eds.), *De-medicalizing misery: Psychiatry, psychology and the human condition* (pp. 1–10). Palgrave Macmillan.

Khan, M., Ilcisin, M., & Saxton, K. (2017). Multifactorial discrimination as a fundamental cause of mental health inequities. *International Journal for Equity in Health, 16*(1), 1–12. https://doi.org/10.1186/s12939-017-0532-z

Laing, M. (2021). Urban Indigenous youth reframing Two-Spirit. *Routledge.* https://doi.org/10.4324/9781003094296

LeFrançois, B. A., Beresford, P., & Russo, J. (2016). Destination Mad Studies. *Intersectionalities: A Global Journal of Social Work Analysis, Research, Polity, and Practice, 5*(3), 1–10. https://journals.library.mun.ca/ojs/index.php/IJ/article/view/1690/1342

LeFrançois, B. A., Menzies, R., & Reaume, G. (2013). Mad matters: A critical reader in Canadian Mad Studies. *Canadian Scholars Press. Doi, 10*(1080/15017419), 2014.

Lewis, B. (2006). *Moving beyond Prozac, DSM, and the new psychiatry: The birth of postpsychiatry*. University of Michigan Press.

McColl, M. A., Adair, B., Davey, S., & Kates, N. (2013). The learning collaborative: An approach to emancipatory research in Disability Studies. *Canadian Journal of Disability Studies, 2*(1), 71–93. https://doi.org/10.15353/cjds.v2i1.71

McIntyre, J., Daley, A., Rutherford, K., & Ross, L. E. (2011). Systems-level barriers in accessing supportive mental health services for sexual and gender minorities: Insights from the provider's perspective. *Canadian Journal of Community Mental Health (revue Canadienne De Santé Mentale Communautaire), 30*(2), 173–186. https://doi.org/10.7870/cjcmh-2011-0023

Meerai, S., Abdillahi, I., & Poole, J. (2016). An introduction to anti-Black sanism. *Intersectionalities: A Global Journal of Social Work Analysis, Research, Polity, and Practice, 5*(3), 18–35. https://journals.library.mun.ca/ojs/index.php/IJ/article/view/1682/1328

Meyer, I. H. (2003). Prejudice, social stress, and mental health in lesbian, gay, and bisexual populations: Conceptual issues and research evidence. *Psychological Bulletin, 129*(5), 674–697. https://doi.org/10.1037/0033-2909.129.5.674

Mills, C. (2014). *Decolonizing global mental health: The psychiatrization of the majority world*. Routledge.

Mills, C. (2017). Global psychiatrization and psychic colonization: The coloniality of global mental health. In M. Morrow & L. Halinka Malcoe (Eds.), *Critical inquiries for social justice in mental health* (pp. 114–137). University of Toronto Press.

Mills, C., & Fernando, S. (2014). Globalising mental health or pathologising the Global South? Mapping the ethics, theory and practice of global mental health. *Disability and the Global South, 1*(2), 188–202. Retrieved August 25, 2021, from https://disabilityglobalsouth.files.wordpress.com/2012/06/dgs-01-02-00.pdf

MindFreedom Ghana. (2019). *Win human rights in mental health*. Retrieved August 19, 2021, from http://www.mindfreedomghana.org

Moosa-Mitha, M. (2005). Situating anti-oppressive theories within critical and difference-centered perspectives. In L. Brown & S. Strega (Eds.), *Research as resistance: Critical, Indigenous, and anti-oppressive approaches* (pp. 38–72). Canadian Scholars Press.

Morrison, M. (2011). Psychological health correlates of perceived discrimination among Canadian gay men and lesbian women. *Canadian Journal of*

Community Mental Health (revue Canadienne De Santé Mentale Communautaire), 30(2), 81–98. https://doi.org/10.7870/cjcmh-2011-0018

Nabbali, E. M. (2013). "Mad" activism and its (Ghanian?) future: A prolegomena to debate. *Trans-Scripts, 3*, 178–201. Retrieved August 19, 2021, from http://sites.uci.edu/transscripts/files/2014/10/2013_03_13.pdf

Piepzna-Samarasinha, L. L. (2018). *Care work: Dreaming disability justice.* Arsenal Pulp Press.

Pilling, M. D. (2013). Invisible identity in the workplace: Intersectional madness and processes of disclosure at work. *Disability Studies Quarterly, 33*(1). https://dsq-sds.org/article/view/3424/3204

Pilling, M. D. (2019). Changing directions or staying the course? Recovery, gender, and sexuality in Canada's mental health strategy. In A. Daley, L. Costa, & P. Beresford (Eds.), *Madness, violence, and power* (pp. 97–114). University of Toronto Press. https://doi.org/10.3138/9781442629981-012

Pilling, M. D., Daley, A., Gibson, M. F., Ross, L. E., & Zaheer, J. (2018). Assessing "insight," determining agency and autonomy: Implicating social identities. In J. M. Kilty & E. Dej (Eds.), *Containing madness: Gender and "psy" in institutional contexts* (pp. 191–213). Palgrave Macmillan. https://doi.org/10.1007/978-3-319-89749-3_9

Poole, J., Jivraj, T., Arslanian, A., Bellows, K., Chiasson, S., Hakimy, H., & Reid, J. (2012). Sanism, "mental health" and social work/education: A review and call to action. *Intersectionalities: A Global Journal of Social Work Analysis, Research, Polity and Practice, 1*(1), 20–36. https://journals.library.mun.ca/ojs/index.php/IJ/article/view/348

Price, M. (2011). *Mad at school: Rhetorics of mental disability and academic life.* University of Michigan Press. https://doi.org/10.3998/mpub.1612837

Rapley, M., Moncrieff, J., & Dillon, J. (2011). Carving nature at its joints? DSM and the medicalization of everyday life. In M. Rapley, J. Moncrieff, & J. Dillon (Eds.), *De-medicalizing misery: Psychiatry, psychology and the human condition* (pp. 1–10). Palgrave Macmillan. https://doi.org/10.1057/978023 0342507_1

Reaume, G. (2006). Mad people's history. *Radical History Review, 94*, 170–182.

Rimke, H. (2016). Introduction—Mental and emotional distress as a social justice issue: Beyond psychocentrism. *Studies in Social Justice, 10*(1), 4–17. https://doi.org/10.26522/ssj.v10i1.1407

Ringer, A., & Holen, M. (2016). "Hell no, they'll think you're mad as a hatter": Illness discourses and their implications for patients in mental health practice. *Health, 20*(2), 161–175. https://doi.org/10.1177/136345931557 4115

Robertson, J., Pote, H., Byrne, A., & Frasquilho, F. (2015). The experiences of lesbian and gay adults on acute mental health wards: Intimate relationship needs and recovery. *Journal of Gay & Lesbian Mental Health, 19*(3), 261–284. https://doi.org/10.1080/19359705.2014.998800

Ross, L. E., Gibson, M. F., Daley, A., Steele, L. S., & Williams, C. C. (2018). In spite of the system: A qualitatively-driven mixed methods analysis of the mental health services experiences of LGBTQ people living in poverty in Ontario Canada. *PLoS ONE, 13*(8), e0201437. https://doi.org/10.1371/jou rnal.pone.0201437

Ross, L. E., Salway, T., Tarasoff, L. A., MacKay, J. M., Hawkins, B. W., & Fehr, C. P. (2018). Prevalence of depression and anxiety among bisexual people compared to gay, lesbian, and heterosexual individuals: A systematic review and meta-analysis. *Journal of Sex Research, 55*(4–5), 435–456. https://doi. org/10.1080/00224499.2017.1387755

Rotondi, N. K., Bauer, G. R., Scanlon, K., Kaay, M., Travers, R., & Travers, A. (2011). Prevalence of and risk and protective factors for depression in female-to-male transgender Ontarians: Trans PULSE Project. *Canadian Journal of Community Mental Health (revue Canadienne De Santé Mentale Communautaire), 30*(2), 135–155. https://doi.org/10.7870/cjcmh-2011-0021

Rotondi, N. K., Bauer, G. R., Travers, R., Travers, A., Scanlon, K., & Kaay, M. (2011). Depression in male-to-female transgender Ontarians: Results from the Trans PULSE project. *Canadian Journal of Community Mental Health (Revue Canadienne de santé mentale communautaire), 30*(2), 113–133. https://doi.org/10.7870/cjcmh-2011-0020

Simeonov, D., Steele, L. S., Anderson, S., & Ross, L. E. (2015). Perceived satisfaction with mental health services in the lesbian, gay, bisexual, transgender, and transsexual communities in Ontario, Canada: An internet-based survey. *Canadian Journal of Community Mental Health, 34*(1), 31–44. https://doi. org/10.7870/cjcmh-2014-037

Snyder, S. N., Pitt, K. A., Shanouda, F., Voronka, J., Reid, J., & Landry, D. (2019). Unlearning through Mad Studies: Disruptive pedagogical praxis. *Curriculum Inquiry, 49*(4), 485–502. https://doi.org/10.1080/03626784. 2019.1664254

Steele, L. S., Daley, A., Curling, D., Gibson, M. F., Green, D. C., Williams, C. C., & Ross, L. E. (2017). LGBT identity, untreated depression, and unmet need for mental health services by sexual minority women and trans-identified people. *Journal of Women's Health, 26*(2), 116–127. https://doi.org/10.1089/jwh.2015.5677

Sutter, M., & Perrin, P. B. (2016). Discrimination, mental health, and suicidal ideation among LGBTQ people of color. *Journal of Counseling Psychology, 63*(1), 98. https://doi.org/10.1037/cou0000126

Szasz, T. (1961). *The myth of mental illness: Foundations of a theory of personal conduct*. Hoeber-Harper. https://doi.org/10.1037/h0046535

Tew, J. (2011). *Social approaches to mental distress*. Palgrave Macmillan. https://doi.org/10.1080/09687599.2012.722410

Tuck, E. (2009). Suspending damage: A letter to communities. *Harvard Educational Review, 79*(3), 409–428. https://pages.ucsd.edu/~rfrank/class_web/ES-114A/Week%204/TuckHEdR79-3.pdf

Williams, C. C., Curling, D., Steele, L. S., Gibson, M. F., Daley, A., Green, D. C., & Ross, L. E. (2017). Depression and discrimination in the lives of women, transgender and gender liminal people in Ontario, Canada. *Health & Social Care in the Community, 25*(3), 1139–1150. https://doi.org/10.1111/hsc.12414

2

Reclaiming the Lunatic Fringe: Toward a Mad-Queer-Trans Lens

There is something queer and trans about madness. The intersections are evident in theoretical overlaps between Queer Studies and Mad Studies, as well as in historical and current activist struggles against psychiatry by LGBTQ people and psychiatric survivors alike. Despite these apparent overlaps, critical scholarly and activist interventions at the intersections of madness, queerness, and transness have been relatively few. This chapter offers some reasons as to why, while also mapping historical and contemporary tensions and overlaps. I begin with a brief discussion of race, sexuality, and gender nonconformance in psychiatric knowledge production and practice. I then trace two genealogical threads of LGBTQ activist resistance to psychiatry in the form of declassification and depathologization struggles and their contemporary scholarly outgrowths. The first genealogical thread is one that has become predominant and describes the origins of a single-issue politic that employed sanist logics in the service of declassifying homosexuality as a mental illness in the DSM, and culminates in contemporary mainstream LGBTQ mental health scholarship. The second genealogical thread is evident in the existence of an intersectional, coalitional politic that was present at the time of declassification struggles but which has

© The Author(s), under exclusive license to Springer Nature
Switzerland AG 2022
M. D. Pilling, *Queer and Trans Madness*,
https://doi.org/10.1007/978-3-030-90413-5_2

been subjugated by the single-issue approach. It is this thread that I argue could blossom into a mad-queer-trans analytic.

This chapter thereby also serves the purpose of explicating the benefits of a mad-queer-trans lens. A broad critique of psychiatry and the biomedical model like the one I employ in this book is sometimes seen as a product of a bygone era and those who espouse such critiques as part of the "lunatic fringe" (Hobson & Leonard, 2001, p. 52). This is meant pejoratively, but perhaps the lunatic fringe can be thought of productively, as a site of queer and trans madness from which to theorize and resist, outside the mainstream. If the centre encompasses sanist, cisnormative, heteronormative, racist, and otherwise oppressive worldviews, is it so bad to be a lunatic on the fringe?[1] What subjugated knowledge might emerge from a site of queer and trans madness? As a preliminary answer to this question, I conclude the chapter with an overview of nascent discussions in the literature that employ a queer mad or a mad queer lens to offer the beginnings of a more cohesive (but not totalizing) narrative of emerging work at the intersection of queer and trans madness. I suggest reclaiming the lunatic fringe as a coalitionary site that resists the relentless co-optation of resistance (Costa et al., 2012) and foregrounds the mutually constitutive character of madness, queerness, and transness as well as intersectional analyses of structural racism, coloniality, sanism, homophobia, transphobia, classism, and other forms of oppression in the biomedical model of mental illness.

Race, Sexuality, and Gender Nonconformance in Psychiatric Knowledge Production and Practice

Psychiatric knowledge production and practice is steeped in white supremacist and colonial racial hierarchies (Fanon, 1961; Fernando, 2010; Gilman, 1985; Joseph, 2014, 2015; Kanani, 2011; Mills, 2017). Ideas about race, civilization, and primitivity informed psychiatric knowledge production as it was first generated in the mid-nineteenth century, with white Europeans and Americans being constructed as "civilized," while racialized people were seen as "uncivilized" and "primitive" (Fernando, 2010, p. 61). Nineteenth-century anthropological and sociological scholars such as Charles Darwin, Herbert Spencer, and Francis Galton theorized that racialized people were at a lesser stage of evolutionary development than white people and that these ideologies were taken on by psychiatry and psychology and continue to inform present day thought (pp. 61–62). Likewise, Joseph (2019) argues that mental health services "have historically been fashioned for Othering, nation building, and segregating purposes that targeted people based on race....These systems produce harm to racialized groups as well as further experiences of racism today as they continue colonial relations and projects" (p. 8). As this also indicates, the notion of racial hierarchy has also been employed by the psy disciplines in regard to Indigenous peoples (Joseph, 2014, 2015; Kanani, 2011; Waldram, 2004; Yellow Bird, 2004). Under the guise of objective science, North American non-Indigenous scholars have constructed Indigenous peoples and cultures as homogenous and static, making essentializing generalizations that ignore individual and cultural differences (Waldram, 2004). Scholarship regarding Indigenous mental health draws heavily on a primitivist discourse that positions Indigenous peoples and cultures as inferior and underdeveloped, yet also utopian, in that they are depicted as "uncontaminated by the pollutants of civilization" (p. 10).

Racist knowledge production about mental health enabled and legitimized a high level of incarceration of racialized and Indigenous people in psychiatric institutions and racist, violent treatment in these facilities (Chunn & Menzies, 1998; Harper, 1988; Hughes, 1992; Jackson, 2002; Joseph, 2014; Kanani, 2011; Menzies & Chunn, 2002; Menzies & Palys, 2006; Roman et al., 2009; Tam, 2013; Vermette, 1988; Yellow Bird, 2004). For example, Yellow Bird (2004) recounts the treatment of Indigenous people in the Hiawatha Asylum for Insane Indians outside Canton, South Dakota, from 1902 to 1933. Indigenous people were often incarcerated indefinitely in the asylum for resisting racist practices and once there were treated violently and inhumanely. Psychiatric institutions, prisons, and residential schools were used in the social control of Indigenous peoples in Canada and the United States in order to displace Indigenous peoples from their lands in the service of land theft by colonial governments (Kanani, 2011). As Nelson (2012) argues, colonial ideologies underpin current mental health care practice: "mental health care in Canada has historically been influenced by the goals and ideologies of colonialism, but it is not often acknowledged that these ideologies persist in the ways that mental health care is delivered today" (p. 5).

Scholars have also pointed to the ways in which anti-Blackness has been foundational to psychiatry (Abdillahi et al., 2017; Gilman, 1985; Hughes, 1992; Jackson, 2002; Meerai et al., 2016; Metzl, 2009). For example, Gilman (1985) contends that there is a longstanding association of Blackness with illness and pathology in Western culture. He points to the ways in which Blackness has long been linked to wildness and madness, citing examples from such varied sources as the Judeo-Christian Bible, Greek medicine, and the work of Mark Twain. Historical psychiatric diagnoses such as dysaesthesia aethiopis during the era of slavery posited that those who had been enslaved would develop a 'condition' that would cause them to destroy property and create havoc while also becoming immune to pain (Fernando, 2010, p. 67). Likewise, drapetomania was a psychiatric 'condition' that was used to pathologize enslaved people who attempted to escape (p. 67). As Gilman (1985) states, "manifestations of the blacks' rejection of the institution of slavery were fitted into the medical model of insanity" (p. 138). Anti-Blackness continues to inform psychiatric practice today (Abdillahi et al., 2017; Meerai et al., 2016; Pilling, 2021). Current diagnoses, while less obviously racist, are still shaped by ideas about racial inferiority (Fernando, 2010, p. 68). Contemporary dominant discourses that position Black people as violent, dangerous, inferior, and alien may contribute to more Black people being diagnosed with schizophrenia, a condition that is "linked" to "alienness" (Fernando, 2010, p. 68; see also Metzl, 2009).

As Somerville (2000) points out, academic work tends to treat the history of race and sexuality as separate and parallel rather than examining the ways in which these histories are entwined. She argues that struggles over the meaning and creation of sexual identity categories occurred at the same time as efforts to define racial categories and that these concurrent struggles were not simply parallel but enmeshed. As she states, "negotiations of the color line…shaped and were shaped by the emergence of notions of sexual identity and the corresponding epistemological uncertainties surrounding them" (p. 3).

In the late nineteenth century, European and North American sexological theories were used to construct 'same-sex' desire and 'cross-gender' characteristics as physical and mental diseases, arguably laying the groundwork for the psychiatric diagnoses of homosexuality, gender identity disorder (GID), and related diagnoses in the DSM. During this period, sexuality increasingly came under the purview of medicine, and sexologists seeking to taxonomize human sexual desires and behaviours constructed new pathological sexual categories such as "the homosexual, pervert, sadist, masochist, and frigid woman" (Bland & Doan, 1998, p. 2). Following Foucault's *History of Sexuality* (1976), which traces the rise of the belief that sexual acts and behaviours are indicative of a certain type of person, many scholars have analyzed sexology to explore this belief. For example, Weeks (1985) argues that under the guise of objective science, sexologists constructed sexuality as the product of nature and created "an elaborate technology of control" (p. 63). Certain sexual practices were defined as pathological and as indicative of an underlying perverse nature. As Felski (1998) also claims, "sexuality was no longer simply a question of particular acts, but was expressed in appearance, personality and even bodily structure" (p. 4). Major sexological texts such as Krafft-Ebing's *Psychopathia Sexualis* (1886) and Ellis's *Sexual Inversion* (1900) are what Somerville (2000) refers to as "hybrid texts," combining theory from "comparative anatomy, with its procedures of bodily measurement, and the nascent techniques of psychology, with its focus on mental development" (p. 19). These categorizations were constructed by sexologists as forms of mental and physical pathology and are thus key in understanding current conceptualizations and intersections of madness, sexuality, gender, and race.

Somerville's (2000) analysis of late-nineteenth- and early-twentieth-century medical literature written by physicians, sexologists, and psychiatrists shows that theories of sexuality depended on racial ideologies. For example, she points to the presence of scientific racism in the works of Krafft-Ebing and Ellis, arguing that the methodologies of racial science provided a model for these sexologists to use in assessing 'sexual inversion.' Race scientists and sexologists also demonstrated gender-related apprehension, focusing on women's bodies as sites of racial and sexual abnormalities. While race scientists focused on the genitalia and reproductive characteristics of African women as markers of racial difference, sexologists saw the bodies of "female inverts" as the "visual key to ranking bodies according to norms of sexuality" (p. 27).

Sexology also reflected the ideologies of eugenics and white supremacy in that homosexuality was seen by sexologists as a form of degeneracy, a concept drawn directly from eugenicist theories. Sexologists concerned about "mixed bodies" (i.e., "inverts" and "intermediate sexes") deployed models already in existence in race science for pathologizing biracial bodies, or "racial hybrids," as examples of the 'degeneration' that took place when 'racial purity' was not maintained (Somerville, 2000, p. 32). Further, sexology made use of psychological theories present in race science in order to cast homosexual desire as a form of perversion: "interracial and same-sex sexuality became analogous within later conceptions of sexual object choice" (p. 37).

The positioning of sexual and gender dissidence as perversions indicative of mental and physical illness gave rise to violent efforts to treat and cure it. Katz (1976) details medical treatments meant to cure lesbians and gays between the years 1884 and 1974 in the United States. These included surgeries such as castration, hysterectomies, vasectomies, oophorectomies, clitoridectomies, and lobotomies, and the administration of drugs such as "hormones, LSD, sexual stimulants, and sexual depressants" (p. 129). Treatment also included hypnosis, electric and chemical shock treatment, aversion therapy, and psychoanalysis and psychotherapy intended to cure homosexuality (p. 129). Likewise, Dickinson (2015) provides a history of electrical and chemical aversion therapies conducted on men receiving treatment for homosexuality and transvestism in Britain between 1935 and 1974. Davison's (2021) transnational account of the history of aversion therapy illuminates the role of the Cold War in shaping research on, and practice of, homosexual aversion therapy in Czechoslovakia in the 1950s and 1960s and in Britain from 1950 to the mid 1970s.

Trans and gender nonconforming people have also been subject to conversion therapy, sometimes called gender-reparative therapy (Winters, 2008). This treatment has often been directed at children because it was found that conversion therapy with adults was unsuccessful (Tosh, 2016, p. 62). Conversion therapy has been associated with suicide among those who have endured it (Salway et al., 2021; Tosh, 2016, p. 64). Some have pointed to the Gender Identity Clinic of the Child Youth and Family Services at the Centre for Addiction and Mental Health in Toronto, Ontario, as a major hub for this approach (Pyne, 2015; Tosh, 2011). After 30 years of operation, this clinic was shut down following an external review completed in 2015 (Zinck & Pignatiello, 2015). However, a recent study confirms that conversion therapy that attempts to change sexual orientation or gender identity remains prevalent in Canada today, especially directed at youth, trans people, immigrants, and racialized people (Salway et al., 2021). Conversion therapy became illegal in Canada when Bill C-4 went into effect on January 7, 2021, though there are ongoing concerns about the efficacy of the ban (Sampson et al., 2022).

Conversion therapy has been directly enabled by the pathologizing of sexual and gender dissidence in the DSM. Homosexuality was included as a disorder in the first (1952) and second (1968) editions of the DSM. The American Psychiatric Association (APA) board of trustees voted to remove it in 1973 in large part because of pressure from gay and lesbian activists (Bayer, 1987). This decision was challenged, leading the APA to hold a referendum on the matter. The majority voted to uphold the decision, but at this time the APA also created the diagnosis of sexual orientation disturbance to pathologize those unhappy with their homosexuality (Stein, 2012, p. 110). This was replaced with ego-dystonic homosexuality (EDH) in the DSM-III (1980), which quickly met with criticism from gay and lesbian activists, and it did not appear in the revised DSM-III-TR (1987). The DSM-III was the first to include the diagnosis of GID for those displaying 'gender variant' behaviour; the diagnosis was required for those seeking transition-related surgeries. Gender identity disorder was changed to gender dysphoria (GD) in DSM-5 (2013) and continues to be the subject of intense debate. While homosexuality is no longer officially diagnosed as a mental illness, GID and GD have been used to pathologize both queer and trans people, as will be discussed below.

LGBTQ Resistance to Psychiatric Diagnoses: A Single-Issue Politic

How have LGBTQ people resisted psychiatric oppression? There are many answers to this question, and much has been written about the struggle to declassify homosexuality and related diagnoses as mental illnesses in the DSM and depathologize trans and gender nonconforming identities and ways of being. In broad strokes, I trace the rise of a single-issue politic employed by some activists at the expense of a coalitionary approach in solidarity with other movements concerned with psychiatric oppression. This is the first of two genealogical threads I discuss in order to show how mainstream LGBTQ resistance to specific diagnoses strengthened psychiatry as a whole and embraced a limited form of empowerment that precluded alliances with others resisting psychiatry.

In some ways, the process of declassifying homosexuality as a mental disorder in the DSM exposed the enculturated character of psychiatry as a whole, revealing the ways in which psychiatric designations of normal and abnormal are intricately tied to predominant social values (Bayer, 1987). Struggles for declassification uncovered the normally obscured enculturated nature of dominant concepts of health and illness. As Bayer (1987) states,

> because concepts of disease and health take form within cultural contexts in ways that often remain hidden from view, the process of change through which certain deviations become labelled as normal or abnormal remains difficult to discern, becoming clear only when historical or social conditions permit the piercing of the veil of "the natural." (p. 13)

However, the larger emancipatory implications of this blow to the foundations of psychiatry and mainstream mental health practice have not been realized, perhaps in part because of what Carr (2019), in her blog post title, calls the "legacies of strategic sanism" employed by activists in declassification struggles. Some lesbian and gay activists who pressured the APA to remove homosexuality and related diagnoses from the DSM employed sanist logic to fight the association between lesbian and gay people and mental illness and assert the healthiness of 'same-sex' desire and relations. Declassification activists aimed to refute previous understandings of homosexuality as a disability or mental illness, thereby distancing gays and lesbians from the associated stigma (Kunzel, 2017, 2018; McRuer, 2006). This was a means of articulating a single-issue politic in order to avoid having to fight the stigma associated with mental illness in addition to the stigma attached to homosexuality (Kunzel, 2017). This was accomplished in part by arguing that psychiatry's understanding of homosexuality was biased because it was based on studies of those who were not characteristic of the "average" homosexual, including those who were incarcerated, those who were already psychiatric patients, and those who were gender nonconforming (Kunzel, 2018). As Kunzel (2018) explains,

> activists' efforts to align gay and lesbian under the norm of health worked to redraw the definitions of the modern gay and lesbian as opposed to the anachronistic homosexual, aligning the modern with a range of linked norms of gender normativity, putative whiteness, economic stability, monogamy, and other forms of belonging, and the latter with sickness, trauma, and mental illness. (p. 468)

The distancing of marginalized groups from disability as a tactic of fighting for equality has a long history. Baynton (2001) points to the history of "women's suffrage, African American freedom, and immigration restriction" as examples of the ways in which oppressed groups have been labelled disabled as a way of justifying oppression and inequality (para. 1). He argues that the efforts to combat marginalization in these three contexts focused on resisting the label of disability, rather than arguing that disability was not grounds for inequality. This suggests that there is "tacit acknowledgement across the political spectrum that when disability is present, inequality is indeed justified" (para. 8).

The declassification of homosexuality is lauded as a great success of the gay liberation movement, ignoring the troubling consequences of single-issue tactics and arguing for equity based on the assertion of mental healthiness and the disavowal of connections between madness and disability, and gay and lesbian people. For example, Minton (2002) describes what he sees as the impact of the APA's decision to declassify homosexuality:

> Thrusting off the straitjacket of sickness empowered gay men and lesbians in two ways. First, it accorded them a sense of personal pride and group solidarity, resources necessary to resist the power of heterosexist ideology....Second, removing the official stamp of illness enabled gay people and their supporters to establish a legitimate foundation for communication (such as gay and lesbian studies). (p. 262)

This is a typical characterization of the benefits of declassifying homosexuality as a mental illness. It suggests that pride, solidarity, and legitimate communication are not possible when one is considered mad or mentally ill, which has been disproved by the efforts of the mad movement, Mad Pride, and mad scholarship. It also reinforces the notion that legitimacy is tied to being seen as sane without acknowledging that this is still problematic for those deemed mad, whether queer or not. In other words, this form of empowerment is at the expense of those who identify as (or who are deemed to be) mentally ill or mad, as well as others who are cast as undesirable or atypical, such as incarcerated, gender nonconforming, and racialized LGBTQ people. As a result of the single-issue approach employed by some activists, the declassification of homosexuality resulted in the remedicalization of madness and the relegitimization of psychiatry more broadly because it allowed psychiatry to "re-establish itself as an impartial expert discourse and a proponent of social diversity at a time when it was being increasingly publicly criticized as moralizing and outmoded" (Lewis, 2016, p. 86). Further, the official removal of homosexuality and ego-dystonic homosexuality (EDH) from the DSM did not put an end to the pathologizing of gays and lesbians.

As Sedgwick (1993) points out, DSM-III, the first DSM to drop the diagnosis of homosexuality, was also the first to list GID. According to her, this new diagnosis continued to pathologize effeminate boys (and to a lesser extent masculine girls), which had previously been subsumed under the diagnosis of homosexuality. Sedgwick claims that the gay movement has been reluctant to protest this diagnosis and its impact on effeminate boys, as it is eager to distance itself from the association of effeminacy with homosexuality and the attending conflation of gender and sexuality. She contends that psychiatry is one of the many institutions that work towards the eradication of gay people and that GID is another tool in the arsenal. Written in 1993, Sedgwick's work does not consider the impact of GID on trans people or the ways in which the trans movement has engaged the diagnosis.

Trans and allied activists and scholars have engaged in different struggles from the gay and lesbian activists of the 1970s because diagnoses such as GID and GD greatly influence access to the technologies of medical transition. These diagnoses have been used as gatekeeping mechanisms to limit the autonomy of trans people who seek surgery and hormones (Butler, 2004; Daley & Mulé, 2014; Lev, 2005; Winters, 2008). Accessing lifesaving transition-related medical procedures comes at the cost of submission to the pathologizing discourse of the psy complex, or as Butler (2004) states, "one must be subjected to a regulatory apparatus…in order to get to the point where something like an exercise in freedom becomes possible" (pp. 90–91). Trans scholars and activists have also critiqued the diagnostic criterion for violently (re)producing and enforcing hegemonic gender norms (Butler, 2004; Daley & Mulé, 2014; Spade, 2006). Echoing Sedgwick (1993), some have shown that GID and GD are used to discipline and regulate queer sexualities as well as non-normative genders in children and adults (Ault & Brzuzy, 2009; Daley & Mulé, 2014; Lev, 2005; Tosh, 2015).[2]

All of these interventions have made important contributions to protecting some trans, non-binary, and queer people from the violence of the psy complex, including conversion therapies, which aim to "cure" children and adults of their 'gender variance' (Tosh, 2015; Winters, 2008). And yet, trans movements have not shown widespread solidarity with mad people or opposed psychiatry more broadly, "perhaps because we have been so keen not to be pathologized, so keen to be accepted as normal, reasonable people" (Fitzpatrick, 2013, p. 31). Fitzpatrick and Voronka (2016) explore tensions and potential alliances between mad and trans movements, arguing that the disciplinary force of psychiatry has been applied to trans and mad people in similar ways. Trans people are "de facto if not self-identified, psychiatric survivors" by virtue of being subject to gender-related (or other) diagnoses. Therefore, they have a natural affinity with non-trans mad people (para. 9). They argue that trans communities should jettison respectability politics and broaden the critique of psychiatry to create alliances with psychiatric survivors and the mad movement, cautioning trans activists not to replicate the sanist tactics and respectability politics employed by some gay and lesbian activists in declassification struggles. As they state, "gay activists mostly have been slow to ask questions about how psychiatrists and psychologists might be treating the other people within their diagnostic empire. Instead the LGB line has mostly been: 'we're not mentally ill, *they* are'" (para. 7; emphasis original). Kirby (2014) further explicates the importance of a broader lens, arguing that "our basic identities are less and less considered a 'mental illness,' but our strategies for surviving are being taken out of context and individualized as 'mental illnesses'" (p. 163).

Thus far, there has not been a widespread show of solidarity or recognition of the overlap and intersections of experience by trans and allied activists and scholars. Similar to the gay and lesbian declassification campaign activists, some have employed the tactic of asserting the existence of mentally healthy trans people as a means to argue for increased autonomy and depathologization. For example, Lev (2005) argues that "approval for medical treatment should not depend on being mentally ill, but on being mentally sound enough to make empowered and healthy decisions regarding one's body and life" (p. 59). This raises the question of who is "mentally sound enough" to exercise decision-making power and make assumptions about the incapacity of those who are mentally ill or mad. It also draws a distinction between "mentally sound" trans people and those who are not, replicating the distancing tactic employed by gay and lesbian activists of the 1970s.

While trans activists no doubt espouse varying positions on the matter, as Lüthi (2016) argues, the distancing tactics employed by depathologization activists have "received the largest media coverage and political support," and as a result, "trans people with experiences of psychiatrization and psychiatric labels other than 'gender identity disorder' or 'gender dysphoria' are written out of the narrative" (p. 135). What about trans people who identify, or are perceived, as mad or mentally ill, who need access to medical technologies of transition? This is an important question, as gatekeeping has been especially strict for variously oppressed trans people, including those who use substances, have a high body mass index, are non-binary, and are not heterosexual. As Kirby (2014) explains, those who have been perceived as mentally ill have often been expected to have their 'condition' "under control" before being allowed to access medical transition (pp. 164–165). This creates a hierarchy whereby surgeries and hormones are more easily accessed based on proximity to oppressive norms.

Ultimately, the narrow focus on the depathologization of specific diagnoses pertaining to sexuality and gender identity is important but does not question the broad medicalization of distress and its impact on 2SLGBTQ people. Furthermore, it abandons queer and trans people who are mad or who are perceived as such and limits opportunities for coalitionary approaches to challenging the psy complex. As Diamond (2017) states,

> choosing to eliminate specific categories of mental illness, while treating emotional and perceptual experiences of the very people who would have been labelled within such categories, separates marginalised people from one another and obscures how systems of power and domination act on our psyches. Contextualising all human experience is a critical step in challenging the pathologisation of queer and trans people. (p. 95)

The next section will begin to trace the genealogical thread of the LGBTQ activism that works towards this broad goal as well as the impact of both threads on contemporary scholarship.

Intersectional Resistance to Psychiatric Oppression

As I have shown, a single-issue politic became predominant in LGBTQ organizing, but there were also activists who engaged in coalitionary resistance. Ferguson (2019) argues that gay and lesbian activism of the 1960s and 70s was intersectional and that these "movements of liberation…were imbricated struggles" (p. 19). He shows that gay liberation had "multidimensional beginnings" in that it was enmeshed with anti-racist, anti-poverty, feminist, and anti-imperialist movements (p. 16). He challenges a linear progress narrative of queer politics, arguing that the current single-issue gay rights framework has misrepresented and erased early intersectional organizing and the activism of trans women of colour such as Silvia Rivera and Marsha P. Johnson, who were involved in multiple intersecting liberation struggles for people of colour, queer, and transgender people. In doing so, he shows how intersectional, coalitionary politics were at the heart of early gay, lesbian, and trans organizing, but have been overtaken by a more conservative, single-issue gay politics that positions critiques of "racism, capitalism, and the state, and their overlaps as outside the normal and practical interests of gay liberation" (p. 9).

While Ferguson does not consider issues of mental illness and disability in any detail, the single-issue politics of declassification activists can usefully be understood as taking place within the multivocal milieu he describes. This resonates with the work of Lewis (2016), who demonstrates that there were conflicting worldviews and activist strategies within gay and lesbian organizing in the 1960s and 70s. As described, the dominant narrative about declassification reflects the values of some gay and lesbian activists who were aligned with psychiatry and employed single-issue politics to distance homosexuality from mental illness. However, Lewis charts the existence of more radical, coalitional gay and lesbian activists, arguing that the more conservative faction was actually at odds with the ethos of the times and other "Left critiques" such as "antiwar, feminist, and black power movements" that critiqued the psy complex (p. 99). These more radical gay and lesbian activists resisted psychiatry more broadly and instead of disavowing madness, explored "homosexuality's continuities with madness, positing both as politically productive models of fractured existence" (p. 101). They embraced a coalitionary politic and recognized the ways in which racism, imperialism, and sexism were imbricated in psychiatric knowledge production (p. 102). Instead of focusing on specific diagnoses, they critiqued psychiatric practices generally, including institutionalization, coercion, and harmful methods such as electro-convulsive therapy (ECT) and psychosurgery (p. 102). Lewis argues that these radical forms of gay and lesbian activism can be seen as a precursor to contemporary conceptions of queer:

> Collectively, these more sweeping refusals of psychiatry constitute an important site of coalition in early LGBT organizing. But they also present a genealogy of antirationalist and anti-identitarian sexual politics that…anticipated the antinormative and deconstructive mandates that are today widely associated with the designation "queer." (p. 87)

Drawing on Lewis's arguments, Daley and Radford (2018) posit that if this more radical faction of gay and lesbian activists can be seen as a genealogy of queer, then the more conservative declassification campaign can be seen as a precursor to the minority stress model and, I would add, contemporary mainstream LGBTQ mental health research more broadly. As described in more detail in Chapter 1, the minority stress model and much of mainstream mental health research claims that LGBTQ people are more vulnerable to mental disorders or have a higher prevalence of mental health problems because of the stigma and discrimination associated with dissident sexualities and genders. This research positions madness as a deficit and as a medical issue requiring medical treatment. As Daley and Radford (2018) argue, "conceivably then, the minority stress model is an outgrowth of the declassification campaign as it inspires the individualising and normalising psychiatric discourses or rather psychocentri[sm]" (p. 294). They go on to state, "the model invokes structural violence as a cause of queer and trans mental and emotional distress; yet, it remains firmly committed to the notion of individual pathology, and thus, continues the well-established pattern of psychiatrising queer and trans people" (p. 295).

This conservative politic has become predominant in the form of mainstream LGBTQ mental health research and has had a strong influence on contemporary LGBTQ scholarly and activist thought in general. While Lewis (2016) may be right in positing early gay and lesbian coalitionary politics as the predecessor to "queer" in terms of anti-identitarian and anti-normative politics, queer activist and scholarly interventions have not always lived up to the coalitionary potential of "queer" in terms of incorporating anti-racism (as demonstrated by queer of color critique), anti-sanism, and explorations of the continuities between madness and queerness. Currently, even those who embrace a queer politic in other respects can be deeply committed to the medicalization of madness, to the point where it can be perceived as offensive to explore other ways of thinking and being. Even within queer and trans communities, structural critiques of the psy complex can be misconstrued as individualizing attacks on the self-identification of those who embrace a mental illness identity or medical responses to distress. This is not to suggest a false binary of being either for or against medicalized models of distress; the reality is much more complex and nuanced. Rather, my point is that psychocentric (Rimke, 2016) ways of thinking have become firmly entrenched within queer and trans communities, sometimes leading to resistance to critiques of the biomedical model and a mad-queer-trans lens, or analytic. As Spandler and Barker (2016) state,

> it is perhaps surprising that communities which think so critically about sexuality and gender often seem not to engage at all with the critical perspectives on mental health....Often in those communities fairly individualistic, essentialist and mainstream understanding of mental health seem to be taken at face value with little awareness of the role of social oppression in distress, or problematising mad/sane binaries....For that reason there's a lot of scope to bring Mad activism into greater dialogue with Queer activism. (para. 42)

As I argue throughout this book, those invested in social justice for 2SLGBTQ people often recognize that the pathologizing of queer and trans identities is problematic, while failing to acknowledge the ways in which biomedical mental health treatment can be damaging. By tracing two genealogical threads, I have offered one possible explanation as to why this is the case, by showing how this mirrors earlier resistance strategies that became predominant by employing sanist logics and single-issue politics. This dynamic has shaped scholarly interventions as well. However, there is an emerging body of literature that considers the intersections of queerness, transness, and madness, which will be discussed in the next section. Perhaps this work can be seen as fulfilling the potential of the coalitional LGBTQ activists.

Toward a Mad-Queer-Trans Lens

LeFrançois and Diamond (2014) argue that queer theorists have largely failed to take up madness or have done so in a way that is "disappointingly individualized, essentialized, and/or othered as 'non-knowledge' or an 'absent space'" (p. 53). Likewise, Mad Studies has been slow to take up issues of heteronormativity, transphobia, and 2SLGBTQ issues, and this book is the first comprehensive application of Mad Studies to queer and trans experiences of mental distress. However, in recent years, some scholars have begun to note similarities between Queer Studies and Mad Studies as modes of inquiry and have produced work at the intersections of queerness, transness, and madness. There are also potential overlaps between Mad Studies and Trans Studies, but these have largely yet to be explored. For this reason, in the following I focus on scholarly works at the intersection of Mad Studies and Queer Studies, but not Trans Studies, though trans is included insofar as Queer Studies often includes (trans)gender analyses.[3] I devote the next section to a brief overview of some of this literature regarding overlap between Queer Studies and Mad Studies as well as scholars employing a queer mad or mad queer lens in order to bring this nascent work together and point to avenues for further study, as well as to highlight the benefits and possibilities of employing a mad-queer-trans lens.

Queer Madness:: Mad Queerness[4]

Perhaps most obviously, both mad and queer are reclaimed slurs and are, therefore, provocative; they make some people angry and they raise questions about who can (or should) use these words and in what context (Spandler & Poursanidou, 2019). Early uses of queer by activists and scholars in the late 1980s and 90s were often anti-identitarian, and queer was seen as impossible to fully define, "a zone of possibilities" (Edelman, 1994, p. 114). Likewise, there has been reluctance to definitively describe what is meant by mad, and Mad Studies is often characterized as emergent and non-prescriptive (Gorman & LeFrançois, 2017). As this suggests, there are similarities between queer and mad as modes of inquiry; they have both been employed as "strategies of critique and resistance" (Spandler & Barker, 2016, para. 10). In other words, both mad and queer have been used as analytics, or lenses, through which to challenge predominant normativities (Spandler, 2017; Spandler & Barker, 2016), as opposed to (or in addition to) as identities. Queer and mad academic projects are both intertwined with associated social movements and grassroots organizing and perhaps because of this, both have struggled with essentialist slippages. As an analytic, queer can be used to denote any body positioned outside of dominant norms (not just 2SLGBTQ bodies). However, it has increasingly been used as an umbrella term and an identity category to describe 2SLGBTQ people. Likewise, mad theory contains a "kernel" of essentialism, or the assumption that there are inherent traits that define mad people (Gorman & LeFrançois, 2017, p. 110).

Queer Studies, Mad Studies, and associated social movements challenge binaries based on colonial constructs of sex, gender, sexuality, and rationality (heterosexual/queer, male/female, sane/mad). In somewhat different ways, they have rejected assimilationist goals, instead embracing difference and working towards creating more space for queer and mad ways of being and knowing rather than aiming to disappear into what is considered 'normal.' Mad Studies employs "subjugated knowledge" to challenge prevailing ideas about mental illness and the psy complex (LeFrançois et al., 2013, p. 14). Similarly, Queer Studies employs the subjugated knowledge of those who transgress gendered, sexualized, and racialized norms and who are positioned as abject or abnormal. Queer Studies explores the ways in which sex, gender, and sexuality are socially constructed and changing over time according to context and culture (Butler, 2004; Fausto-Sterling 2000; Ferguson, 2004). Likewise, Mad Studies considers the ways in which madness is socially constructed (Spandler & Barker, 2016).[5]

Both have been critiqued for a lack of consideration of race, colonialism, and experiences of racialized and Indigenous peoples (Abdillahi et al., 2017; Cohen, 2005; Driskill, 2010; Driskill et al., 2011; Ferguson, 2004; Gorman, 2013; Johnson et al., 2005; Joseph, 2015, 2019; Morgenson, 2010; Muñoz, 1999; Pickens, 2019; Tam, 2013). Queer of colour critique has made important interventions in Queer Studies, pointing to the ways in which it has centred whiteness, excluded critical analyses of race and racism, and overlooked coalitionary potential (Cohen, 2005; Ferguson, 2004; Johnson et al., 2005; Muñoz, 1999). Likewise, scholars have pointed to the necessity of paying attention to colonialism, Indigeneity, and two-spirit experiences in Queer Studies (Driskill, 2010; Driskill et al., 2011; Morgenson, 2010, 2011; Smith, 2010) as well as the lack of attention to sex, gender, and sexuality as colonial constructs employed as tools of colonization (Picq & Tikuna, 2019). Similar interventions have been made in Mad Studies, with some scholars pointing to the lack of attention being paid to the ways in which racism, colonialism, and Eurocentrism shape psychiatric knowledge and practice (Gorman, 2013; Joseph, 2015, 2019), the mutually constitutive nature of sanism/ableism and anti-Blackness (Abdillahi et al., 2017; Meerai et al., 2016; Pickens, 2019), and the problematic ways in which non-Indigenous Mad Studies scholars have employed colonialism as a metaphor for psychiatric violence (Gorman et al., 2013; Mills, 2017). As this indicates, a mad-queer-trans lens must decentre whiteness and include strong analyses of the co-constitutive nature of racism, colonialism, sanism/ableism, heteronormativity, transphobia, classism, and other forms of oppression. The following will highlight some emerging work that employs a queer mad or mad queer lens.

Queer Madness

LeFrançois and Diamond (2014) and Diamond (2017) employ queer theory to explore the social construction of psychiatric diagnoses and demonstrate that there is no fixed, or essential, referent point for states of mental health or illness. Similar to how queer theorists have shown that sexuality and gender categories are fluid and change in meaning across time and culture, this work argues that psychiatric diagnoses are fluid and change according to cultural and historical context. LeFrançois and Diamond (2014) emphasize that any queering of psychiatry must also consider "deeply embedded structural racism and institutionalized white privilege…as organizing principles" (p. 40). While LeFrançois and Diamond (2014) apply a queer lens to the psychiatrization of children,

Diamond (2017) emphasizes the importance of understanding queer and trans experiences of distress within the larger context of structural oppression and of challenging the psychiatrizing of distress experienced by queer and trans people, rather than focusing on specific diagnoses that target non-normative genders and sexualities. As she states, "a change in diagnosis without a change in the flawed foundational organisation of psy-theories and services does not move us closer to better serving queer and trans people" (p. 96).

Morrigan (2017) and Rowe and Chávez (2011) explore queer mad world-making. Morrigan "maddens" queer temporalities by considering the ways in which experiences of trauma shape relationships to time, arguing that "the queer time travel of trauma can be a means of queer, mad, world-making" (p. 57). Rowe and Chavez employ a "queer performativity of madness" to explore the work of queer feminist Valerie Solanas, arguing that this approach allows for visions of "nonnormative worlds beyond what rational engagements with politics and theory provide" (p. 282). Queer theory has also been used alongside critical race theory to challenge the mad/sane binary, exploring the ways in which the "mad border body serves as a counter-narrative for madness and sanity" (Kafai, 2013, para. 2). Using Anzaldua's concept of the borderland and Zita's term "border body," Kafai challenges essentialist binary identity categories, reimagining madness as a place of "in-betweeness."

Mad Queerness

Some scholars have employed a combined queer and mad lens, such as Daley and Radford (2018). They apply a mad queer abolitionist lens to queer and trans incarceration distress to challenge an LGBTQ-rights approach and the minority stress model. This mad queer abolitionist lens is used to intervene in the individualizing and pathologizing of queer and trans responses to the structural violence of heteronormativity and cisnormativity as they intersect with white supremacy and institutionalized racism in the prison system. In my own work, I have applied an intersectional Mad Studies lens to mad, queer, and trans disclosures in the workplace (Pilling, 2013) and employed a mad critique of the Mental

Health Commission of Canada's mental health strategy as it pertains to 2SLGBTQ people (Pilling, 2019).

White Supremacy and Heteronormativity in Psychiatric Chart Documentation Practices

Some scholars have employed a mad lens to "study up" (Harding & Norberg, 2005), turning the gaze on the psychiatric institution to expose the heteronormative, classed, and white supremacist logics of psychiatric chart documentation practices. For example, Metzl et al. (2016) demonstrate a white, heterosexist bias within psychiatric charting. They argue that while the charts they studied contained no explicit diagnosing of homosexuality, documentation showed that "the gendered politics of diagnosis were anything but value-free, in as much as clinical interactions...still held white heteronormativity as mental health and treated it as such" (p. 254). Similarly, Pilling et al.'s (2018) analysis of psychiatric inpatient charting shows that the psychiatric construct of "insight" is used to delegitimize disagreement with the biomedical model, particularly for those who are marginalized by heterosexism, racism, classism, and other forms of structural oppression. Likewise, I explore the confluence of rape culture, sanism, and anti-Blackness in psychiatric inpatient documentation regarding sexual violence (Pilling, 2021). Daley and Ross (2018) use Rimke's (2016) concept of psychocentrism to analyze the erasure of queer madness and 'same-sex' intimate partner violence in psychiatric inpatient charting, and Ross and Costa (2021) explore the psychiatrization of bisexual people in psychiatric inpatient charting.

Mad Queer Considerations of Care

The thorny issue of care is one around which queer and mad analyses converge. For example, Horncastle (2018) writes at the intersections "of queer poetics, mad studies and phenomenological theories of suicidality" to investigate the meaning of care in hospital and medical settings (p. 383). The focus on care has clear connections to a Disability Justice framework (see, for example, Piepzna-Samarasinha, 2018). For example, Johnk and Khan's (2019) written performance piece draws on the authors' subjugated knowledge as "disabled, Mad and/or neurodivergent people" and on "women of color feminisms, queer and trans of color critiques, Two-Spirit critiques, and Disability Justice" to expose and resist the ways in which pathologization is reconfigured as care within the "Medical Industrial Complex" (p. 27). Likewise, Eales and Peers (2020) draw on Disability Justice to highlight both the promise and the violence of care at the intersections of capitalism, colonialism, white supremacy, heterosexism, and cisnormativity. Their "creative duo-ethnography" uses a mad, queer, crip lens to explore the notion of care, exposing the violence that can be enacted through care and the importance and possibilities of "cripping care" within mad, disabled, and queer communities.

This overview indicates that there are multiple ways of employing a mad-queer-trans lens, including those that have yet to be explored. While some scholars apply queer theory or Queer Studies to issues of madness, others apply Mad Studies to queer and trans experiences, and consider how madness, queerness, and transness are mutually constitutive. A mad-queer-trans lens is not prescriptive and can foreground various contextual aspects of mutually constitutive systems of power including white supremacy, colonialism, heteropatriarchy, and cisnormativity.

This overview is not meant to be an exhaustive account of all relevant literature and overlaps between madness, queerness, and transness. For example, the literature on queer and trans abolition is relevant to considerations of resisting carcerality in psychiatric contexts (Ben-Moshe, 2020; Ben-Moshe et al., 2014, 2015; Richie, 2005; Smith & Stanley, 2015; Stanley & Spade, 2012; Vitulli, 2013). As the first half of this chapter indicates, there is also a body of work that looks at mad, queer, and trans considerations pertaining to desclassification struggles and historical and contemporary LGBTQ organizing (Carr, 2019; Fitzpatrick, 2013; Fitzpatrick & Voronka, 2016; Kirby, 2014; Kunzel, 2017, 2018; Lüthi, 2016; Tosh, 2015) including the role of queer psy professionals in resisting pathologization and dominant social norms (Hubbard, 2020; Spandler & Carr, 2021). Some of the other relevant areas include crip theory (Kafer, 2013; McRuer, 2006; Samuels, 2003), crip of color critique (Kim, 2017; Kim & Schalk, 2021), Disability Justice (Bernes, 2015; Mingus, n.d.; Piepzna-Samarasinha, 2018), work at the inter-sections of transness and disability (Baril, 2015; Clare, 2017; George, 2019; Slater & Liddiard, 2018), and emerging literature in neurodiver-sity (Hart, 2020; McWade et al., 2015) and neuroqueer (Egner, 2019; Walker, 2015). All of these areas of study point toward productive overlaps between queerness, madness, and transness.

In this chapter I have begun to address what is queer and trans about madness and offer a partial explanation for some of the reasons why coalitionary, intersectional approaches to psychiatric oppression have not been predominant in mainstream LGBTQ organizing and scholarship. There are no doubt other considerations that could provide a more fulsome answer to this question, including analyses of the history of the anti-psychiatry movement and other movements for social justice. I have shown that mad-queer-trans analytics lend themselves to a coali-tionary stance instead of limited empowerment for some at the expense of others. This subjugated knowledge, which is sometimes perceived as coming from a "lunatic fringe," may be harder to co-opt given it is less compatible with mainstream, rights-based, and single-issue approaches. It can illuminate and resist predominant normativities, look more critically at what constitutes psychiatric treatment, and examine the biomedical model of mental illness more broadly while foregrounding intersectional analyses of structural homophobia, transphobia, racism, coloniality, sanism, classism, and other forms of oppression. The next chapter will draw on participant narratives from the Queer and Trans Madness study to present a critique of the biomedical model and high-light the benefits of a mad-queer-trans lens in understanding 2SLGBTQ experiences of mental distress.

Notes

1. There are no doubt contexts in which the answer to this question is yes. This question is not meant to minimize the very real harms that are inflicted on marginalized groups.

2. For a detailed history of the pathologizing of gender nonconformance and trans activism in response to the diagnoses of GID and GD. See Tosh (2015).
3. The relationship between queer theory and trans experience is fraught. See Stryker (2004).
4. This subheading is a nod to Theri Alyce Pickens's (2019) Black Madness:: Mad Blackness, which argues that "in an ideological construct of white supremacy, Blackness is considered synonymous with madness or the prerequisite for creating madness" (p. 4) and is a reminder that focusing on queerness and transness should not preclude the ways in which madness is also racialized.
5. For a detailed description of the differences and similarities between Mad Studies and Queer Studies, see Spandler and Barker (2016).

References

Abdillahi, I., Meerai, S., & Poole, J. (2017). When the suffering is compounded: Towards anti-Black sanism. In S. Wehbi & H. Parada (Eds.), *Reimagining anti-oppression social work practice* (pp. 109–122). Canadian Scholars Press.

Ault, A., & Brzuzy, S. (2009). Removing gender identity disorder from the *Diagnostic and Statistical Manual of Mental Disorders*: A call for action. *Social Work, 54*(2), 187–189. https://doi.org/10.1093/sw/54.2.187

Baril, A. (2015). Transness as debility: Rethinking intersections between trans and disabled embodiments. *Feminist Review, 111*(1), 59–74. https://doi.org/10.1057/fr.2015.21

Bayer, R. (1987). *Homosexuality and American psychiatry*. Princeton University Press.

Baynton, D. C. (2001). *Disability and the justification of inequality in American history*. Disability History Museum. Retrieved August 19, 2021, from https://www.disabilitymuseum.org/dhm/edu/essay.html?id=70

Ben-Moshe, L. (2020). *Decarcerating disability: Deinstitutionalization and prison abolition*. University of Minnesota Press. https://doi.org/10.5749/j.ctv10vm2vw

Ben-Moshe, L., Chapman, C., & Carey, A. C. (2014). *Disability incarcerated: Imprisonment and disability in the United States and Canada*. Palgrave Macmillan. https://doi.org/10.1057/9781137388476

Ben-Moshe, L., Gossett, C., Mitchell, N., & Stanley, E. A. (2015). Critical theory, queer resistance, and the ends of capture. In G. Adelsberg, L. Guenther, & S. Zeman (Eds.), *Death and other penalties: Philosophy in a time of mass incarceration* (pp. 266–296). Fordham University Press.

Bernes, P. (2015). *Disability justice—A working draft by Patty Berne*. Retrieved August 19, 2021, from https://www.sinsinvalid.org/blog/disability-justice-a-working-draft-by-patty-berne

Bland, L., & Doan, L. (1998). *Sexology uncensored: The documents of sexual science*. University of Chicago Press.

Butler, J. (2004). *Undoing gender*. Routledge.

Carr, S. (2019, June 23). Madness, sexuality, and legacies of strategic sanism: *Mad in America*. Retrieved August 19, 2021, from https://www.madinamerica.com/2019/06/madness-sexuality-strategic-sanism/

Chunn, D. E., & Menzies, R. (1998). Out of mind, out of law: The regulation of criminally insane women inside British Columbia's public mental hospitals, 1888–1973. *Canadian Journal of Women and Law, 10*, 306–337. https://eugenicsarchive.ca/discover/tree/525e043ac6813a5469000002

Clare, E. (2017). Brilliant imperfection: Grappling with cure. *Duke University Press*. https://doi.org/10.1215/9780822373520

Cohen, C. J. (2005). Punks, bulldaggers, and welfare queens: The radical potential of queer politics? In P. Johnson & M. Henderson (Eds.), *Black Queer Studies* (pp. 21–51). Duke University Press.

Costa, L., Voronka, J., Landry, D., Reid, J., Mcfarlane, B., Reville, D., & Church, K. (2012). "Recovering our stories": A small act of resistance. *Studies in Social Justice, 6*(1), 85–101. https://doi.org/10.26522/ssj.v6i1.1070

Daley, A., & Mulé, N. J. (2014). LGBTQs and the DSM-5: A critical queer response. *Journal of Homosexuality, 61*(9), 1288–1312. https://doi.org/10.1080/00918369.2014.926766

Daley, A., & Radford, K. (2018). Queer and trans incarceration distress: Considerations from a Mad Queer abolitionist perspective. In A. Mills & K. Kendall (Eds.), *Mental health in prisons* (pp. 285–307). Palgrave Macmillan. https://doi.org/10.1007/978-3-319-94090-8_12

Daley, A., & Ross, L. E. (2018). Uncovering the heteronormative order of the psychiatric institution: A queer reading of chart documentation and language use. In J. Kilty & E. Dej (Eds.), *Containing madness: Gender and "psy" in institutional contexts* (pp. 169–190). Palgrave Macmillan. https://doi.org/10.1007/978-3-319-89749-3_8

Davison, K. (2021). Cold War Pavlov: Homosexual aversion therapy in the 1960s. *History of the Human Sciences, 34*(1), 89–119.

Diamond, S. (2017). Trapped in change: Using queer theory to examine the progress of psy-theories and interventions with sexuality and gender. In B. M. Z. Cohen (Ed.), *Routledge international handbook of critical mental health* (pp. 89–97). Routledge. https://doi.org/10.4324/9781315399584-12

Dickinson, T. (2015). *'Curing queers': Mental nurses and their patients, 1935–74.* Manchester University Press.

Driskill, Q. L. (2010). Doubleweaving two-spirit critiques: Building alliances between Native and Queer Studies. *GLQ: A Journal of Lesbian and Gay Studies, 16*(1–2), 69–92. https://doi.org/10.1215/10642684-2009-013

Driskill, Q. L., Finley C., Gilley, B. J., & Morgensen S. L. (2011). The revolution is for everyone: Imagining an emancipatory future through queer Indigenous critical theories. In Q. L. Driskill, C. Finley, Gilley, B. J., & S. L. Morgensen (Eds.), *Queer Indigenous Studies: Critical interventions in theory, politics, and literature* (pp. 211–221). University of Arizona Press. http://web.colby.edu/queer-theory-fall18/files/2018/09/Queer-indigenous-Studies.pdf

Eales, L., & Peers, D. (2020). Care haunts, hurts, heals: The promiscuous poetics of queer crip Mad care. *Journal of Lesbian Studies, 25*(3), 1–19. https://doi.org/10.1080/10894160.2020.1778849

Edelman, L. (1994). *Homographesis: Essays in gay literary and cultural theory.* Routledge.

Egner, J. E. (2019). "The disability rights community was never mine": Neuroqueer disidentification. *Gender & Society, 33*(1), 123–147. https://doi.org/10.1177/0891243218803284

Fanon, F. (1961). *The wretched of the earth.* Présence Africaine.

Fausto-Sterling, A. (2000). *Sexing the body: Gender politics and the construction of sexuality.* Basic Books.

Felski, R. (1998). Introduction. In L. Bland & L. Doan (Eds.), *Sexology in culture* (pp. 116–133). University of Chicago Press.

Ferguson, R. A. (2004). *Aberrations in Black: Toward a queer of color critique.* University of Minnesota Press.

Ferguson, R. A. (2019). *One-dimensional queer.* Polity Press.

Fernando, S. (2010). *Mental health, race and culture.* Palgrave Macmillan. https://doi.org/10.1007/978-1-137-01368-2_2

Fitzpatrick, C. (2013). Dear Mad Pride, with gratitude. *Asylum, 20*(4), 30–31. https://asylummagazine.org/wp-content/uploads/2019/09/Asylum-20.4-2013-Mad-in-Toronto_compressed.pdf

Fitzpatrick, C., & Voronka, J. (2016). Trans activists, don't throw mad people under the bus! *Feministing*. Retrieved August 19, 2021, from http://feministing.com/2016/02/10/trans-activists-dont-throw-mad-people-under-the-bus/

Foucault, M. (1976). *The history of sexuality* (Vol. I). Random House.

George, D. (2019). Disabling transgender: Identity-politics navigating mentalism and law. *Journal of Ethics in Mental Health, 10*, 1–8. https://jemh.ca/issues/v9/documents/JEMH%20Inclusion%20xii.pdf

Gilman, S. (1985). *Difference and pathology: Stereotypes of sexuality, race, and madness*. Cornell University Press.

Gorman, R. (2013). Thinking through race, class, and mad identity politics. In B. A. LeFrançois, R. Menzies, & G. Reaume (Eds.), *Mad matters: A critical reader in Canadian Mad Studies* (pp. 269–280). Canadian Scholars Press.

Gorman, R., & LeFrançois, B. A. (2017). Mad Studies. In *Routledge international handbook of critical mental health* (pp. 107–114). Routledge.

Gorman, R., Saini, A., Tam, L., Udegbe, O., & Usar, O. (2013). Mad people of color—A manifesto, *Asylum, 20*(4), 27. Retrieved June 10, 2021, from https://asylummagazine.org/2013/12/mad-people-of-color-a-manifesto-by-rachel-gorman-annu-saini-louise-tam-onyinyechukwu-udegbe-onar-usar/

Harding, S., & Norberg, K. (2005). New feminist approaches to social science methodologies: An introduction. *Signs, 30*(4), 2009–2015. https://doi.org/10.1086/428420

Harper, V. (1988). Them crazy Indians. In B. Burstow & D. Weitz (Eds.), *Shrink resistant: The struggle against psychiatry in Canada* (pp. 121–125). New Star Books.

Hart, A. (2020). A new alliance? The hearing voices movement and neurodiversity. In H. Bertilsdotter Rosqvist, N. Chown, & A. Stenning (Eds.), *Neurodiversity Studies: A new critical paradigm* (pp. 221–225). Routledge. https://doi.org/10.4324/9780429322297-22

Hobson, J. A., & Leonard, J. (2001). *Out of its mind: Psychiatry in crisis: A call for reform*. Basic Books.

Horncastle, J. (2018). Practicing care: Queer vulnerability in the hospital. *Social Identities, 24*(3), 383–394. https://doi.org/10.1080/13504630.2017.1387038

Hubbard, K. (2020). *Queer ink: a blotted history towards liberation*. Routledge.

Hughes, J. S. (1992). Labeling and treating Black mental illness in Alabama, 1861–1910. *Journal of Southern History, 58*(3), 435–460. https://doi.org/10.2307/2210163

Jackson, V. (2002). In our own voice: African-American stories of oppression, survival and recovery in mental health systems. *International Journal of Narrative Therapy & Community Work, 2002*(2), 11–31. https://dulwichce ntre.com.au/wp-content/uploads/2014/08/In_Our_Own_Voice_African_A merican_stories_of_oppression_survival_and_recovery_in_mental_health_ systems.pdf

Johnk, L., & Khan, S. A. (2019). "Cripping the fuck out": A Queer Crip Mad manifesta against the medical industrial complex. *Feral Feminisms, 9*, 27–38. https://feralfeminisms.com/wp-content/uploads/2019/12/4-Johnk-and-Khan.pdf

Johnson, E. P., Henderson, M. G., Holland, S. P., & Cohen, C. J. (2005). *Black Queer Studies: A critical anthology*. Duke University Press. https://doi. org/10.1515/9780822387220

Joseph, A. J. (2014). A prescription for violence: The legacy of colonization in contemporary forensic mental health and the production of difference. *Critical Criminology, 22*(2), 273–292. https://link.springer.com/article/10. 1007/s10612-013-9208-1

Joseph, A. J. (2015). The necessity of an attention to Eurocentrism and colonial technologies: An addition to critical mental health literature. *Disability & Society, 30*(7), 1021–1041. https://doi.org/10.1080/09687599. 2015.1067187

Joseph, A. J. (2019). Constituting "lived experience" discourses in mental health: The ethics of racialized identification/representation and the erasure of intergeneration colonial violence. *Journal of Ethics in Mental Health, 10*, 1–23. https://jemh.ca/issues/v9/documents/JEMH%20Inclusion%20i.pdf

Kafai, S. (2013). The mad border body: A political in-betweeness. *Disability Studies Quarterly, 33*(1). https://dsq-sds.org/article/view/3438/3199

Kafer, A. (2013). *Feminist, Queer*. Indiana University Press.

Kanani, N. (2011). Race and madness: Locating the experiences of racialized people with psychiatric histories in Canada and the United States. *Critical Disability Discourse, 3*, 1–14. https://cdd.journals.yorku.ca/index.php/cdd/ article/view/31564

Katz, J. N. (1976). *Gay American history: Lesbians and gay men in the U.S.A., a documentary anthology*. Crowell.

Kim, J. B. (2017). Toward a crip-of-color critique: Thinking with Minich's "enabling whom?" *Lateral, 6*(1). https://doi.org/10.25158/L6.1.14

Kim, J. B., & Schalk, S. (2021). Reclaiming the radical politics of self-care: A crip-of-color critique. *South Atlantic Quarterly, 120*(2), 325–342. Retrieved

August 20, 2021, from http://samischalk.com/wp-content/uploads/2021/05/Schalk_Black-Disability-Gone-Viral_CLA-Journal-2021.pdf

Kirby, A. (2014). Trans jeopardy/Trans resistance: Shaindl Diamond interviews Ambrose Kirby. In B. Burstow, B. LeFrançois, & S. Diamond (Eds.), *Psychiatry disrupted: Theorizing resistance and crafting the (r)evolution* (pp. 163–176). McGill-Queen's University Press.

Kunzel, R. (2017). Queer history, mad history, and the politics of health. *American Quarterly, 69*(2), 315–319. https://doi.org/10.1353/aq.2017.0026

Kunzel, R. (2018). The rise of gay rights and the disavowal of disability in the United States. In M. Rembis, C Kudlick, & K. E. Nielsen (Eds.), *The Oxford handbook of disability history* (pp. 459–476). https://doi.org/10.1093/oxfordhb/9780190234959.013.27

LeFrançois, B. A., & Diamond, S. (2014). Queering the sociology of diagnosis: Children and the constituting of "mentally ill" subjects. *Journal of Critical Anti-Oppressive Social Inquiry, 1*(1). https://caos.library.ryerson.ca/index.php/caos/article/view/98

LeFrançois, B. A., Menzies, R., & Reaume, G. (2013). *Mad matters: A critical reader in Canadian Mad Studies*. Canadian Scholars Press. https://doi.org/10.1080/15017419.2014

Lev, A. I. (2005). Disordering gender identity: Gender identity disorder in the DSM-IV-TR. *Journal of Psychology and Human Sexuality, 17*(3/4), 35–69. https://doi.org/10.1300/J056v17n03_03

Lewis, A. J. (2016). "We are certain of our own insanity": Antipsychiatry and the gay liberation movement, 1968–1980. *Journal of the History of Sexuality, 25*(1), 83–113. https://doi.org/10.7560/jhs25104

Lüthi, E. H. (2016). Relocating Mad_Trans re_presentations within an intersectional framework. *Intersectionalities: A Global Journal of Social Work Analysis, Research, Polity, and Practice, 5*(3), 130–150. https://journals.library.mun.ca/ojs/index.php/IJ/article/view/1603

McRuer, R. (2006). *Crip theory: Cultural signs of queerness and disability* (Vol. 9). NYU Press.

McWade, B., Milton, D., & Beresford, P. (2015). Mad Studies and neurodiversity: A dialogue. *Disability & Society, 30*(2), 305–309. https://doi.org/10.1080/09687599.2014.1000512

Meerai, S., Abdillahi, I., & Poole, J. (2016). An introduction to anti-Black sanism. *Intersectionalities: A Global Journal of Social Work Analysis, Research, Polity, and Practice, 5*(3), 18–35. https://journals.library.mun.ca/ojs/index.php/IJ/article/view/1682

Menzies, R., & Chunn, D. E. (2002). Race, reason, and regulation: British Columbia's mass exile of Chinese "lunatics" aboard the Empress of Russia, 9 February 1935. In J. P. S. McLaren, R. Menzies, & D. E. Chunn (Eds.), *Regulating lives: Historical essays on the state, society, the individual, and the law* (pp. 196–230). UBC Press.

Menzies, R., & Palys, T. (2006). Turbulent spirits: Aboriginal patients in the British Columbia psychiatric system, 1879–1950. In J. Moran & D. Wright (Eds.), *Mental health and Canadian society: Historical perspectives* (pp. 149–175). McGill-Queen's University Press.

Metzl, J. M. (2009). *The protest psychosis: How schizophrenia became a Black disease.* Beacon Press.

Metzl, J. M., McClelland, S. I., & Bergner, E. (2016). Conflations of marital status and sanity: Implicit heterosexist bias in psychiatric diagnosis in physician-dictated charts at a Midwestern medical center. *Yale Journal of Biology and Medicine, 89*(2), 247–254. https://www.ncbi.nlm.nih.gov/pmc/articles/PMC4918875/

Mills, C. (2017). Global psychiatrization and psychic colonization: The coloniality of global mental health. In M. Morrow & L. Halinka Malcoe (Eds.), *Critical inquiries for social justice in mental health* (pp. 114–137). University of Toronto Press.

Mingus, M. (n.d.). *Leaving evidence.* Retrieved August 20, 2021, from https://leavingevidence.wordpress.com/about-2/

Minton, H. (2002). *Departing from deviance: A history of homosexual rights and emancipatory science in America.* University of Chicago Press.

Morgensen, S. L. (2010). Settler homonationalism: Theorizing settler colonialism within queer modernities. *GLQ: A Journal of Lesbian and Gay Studies, 16*(1–2), 105–131. https://doi.org/10.1215/10642684-2009-015

Morgensen, S. L. (2011). Unsettling queer politics. In Q. L. Driskill, C. Finley, B. J. Gilley, & S. L. Morgensen (Eds.), *Queer Indigenous Studies: Critical interventions in theory, politics, and literature* (pp. 132–52). University of Arizona Press. http://web.colby.edu/queer-theory-fall18/files/2018/09/Queer-indigenous-Studies.pdf

Morrigan, C. (2017). Trauma time: The queer temporalities of the traumatized mind. *Somatechnics, 7*(1), 50–58. 10.3366/soma.2017.0205

Muñoz, J. E. (1999). *Disidentifications: Queers of color and the performance of politics.* University of Minnesota Press.

Nelson, S. (2012). *Challenging hidden assumptions: Colonial norms as determinants of Aboriginal mental health.* National Collaborating Centre for

Aboriginal Health. Retrieved August 21, 2021, https://www.ccnsa-nccah.ca/docs/determinants/FS-ColonialNorms-Nelson-EN.pdf

Pickens, T. A. (2019). *Black Madness: Mad Blackness*. Duke University Press.

Picq, M. L., & Tikuna, J. O. S. I. (2019). Indigenous sexualities: Resisting conquest and translation. In C. Cottet & M. L. Picq (Eds.), *Sexuality and translation in world politics*. E-International Relations. Retrieved August 20, 2021, from https://www.e-ir.info/2019/08/20/indigenous-sexualities-resisting-conquest-and-translation/

Piepzna-Samarasinha, L. L. (2018). *Care work: Dreaming disability justice*. Arsenal Pulp Press.

Pilling, M. D. (2013). Invisible identity in the workplace: Intersectional madness and processes of disclosure at work. *Disability Studies Quarterly, 33*(1). https://dsq-sds.org/article/view/3424/3204

Pilling, M. D. (2019). Changing directions or staying the course? Recovery, gender, and sexuality in Canada's mental health strategy. In A. Daley, L. Costa, & P. Beresford (Eds.), *Madness, violence, and power* (pp. 97–114). University of Toronto Press. https://doi.org/10.3138/9781442629981-012

Pilling, M. D. (2021). Sexual violence and psychosis: Intersections of rape culture, sanism, and anti-Black sanism in psychiatric inpatient chart documentation. In A. Daley & M. D. Pilling (Eds.), *Interrogating psychiatric narratives of madness: Documented lives* (pp. 137–164). Palgrave Macmillan.

Pilling, M. D., Daley, A., Gibson, M. F., Ross, L. E., & Zaheer, J. (2018). Assessing "insight," determining agency and autonomy: Implicating social identities. In J. Kilty & E. Dej (Eds.), *Containing madness: Gender and "psy" in institutional contexts* (pp. 191–213). Palgrave Macmillan. https://doi.org/10.1007/978-3-319-89749-3_9

Pyne, J. (2015, December 17). Discredited treatment of trans kids at CAMH shouldn't shock us. *Toronto Star*. Retrieved August 20, 2021, from https://www.thestar.com/opinion/commentary/2015/12/17/discredited-treatment-of-trans-kids-at-camh-shouldnt-shock-us.html

Richie, B. (2005). Queering antiprison work: African American lesbians in the juvenile justice system. In J. Sudbury (Ed.), *Global lockdown: Race, gender, and the prison-industrial complex* (pp. 73–85). Routledge.

Rimke, H. (2016). Introduction—Mental and emotional distress as a social justice issue: Beyond psychocentrism. *Studies in Social Justice, 10*(1), 4–17. https://doi.org/10.26522/ssj.v10i1.1407

Roman, L. G., Brown, S., Noble, S., Wainer, R., & Young, A. E. (2009). No time for nostalgia! Asylum-making, medicalized colonialism in British

Columbia (1859–97) and artistic praxis for social transformation. *International Journal of Qualitative Studies in Education, 22*(1), 17–63. https://doi.org/10.1080/09518390802581919

Ross, L. E., & Costa, L. (2021). "Slighted and unheard": The psychiatrization of bisexuality. In A. Daley & M. D. Pilling (Eds.), *Interrogating psychiatric narratives of madness: Documented lives* (pp. 87–110). Palgrave Macmillan.

Rowe, D. D., & Chávez, K. R. (2011). Valerie Solanas and the queer performativity of madness. *Cultural Studies? Critical Methodologies, 11*(3), 274–284. https://doi.org/10.1177/1532708611409544

Salway, T., Juwono, S., Klassen, B., Ferlatte, O., Ablona, A., Pruden, H., Morgan, J., Kwag, M., Card, K., Knight, R., & Lachowsky, N. J. (2021). Experiences with sexual orientation and gender identity conversion therapy practices among sexual minority men in Canada, 2019–2020. *PLoS One, 16*(6), e0252539. https://doi.org/10.1371/journal.pone.0252539

Sampson, A., Cowley, J., Szeto, E., & Tomlinson, A. (2022). Conversion therapy is illegal in Canada. But some U.S. life coaches are offering it to Canadians online. https://www.cbc.ca/news/canada/marketplace-life-coach-conversion-therapy-1.6369104

Samuels, E. J. (2003). My body, my closet: Invisible disability and the limits of coming-out discourse. *GLQ: A Journal of Lesbian and Gay Studies, 9*(1), 233–255. https://doi.org/10.1215/10642684-9-1-2-233

Sedgwick, E. K. (1993). *Tendencies.* Duke University Press.

Spandler, H., & Poursanidou, D. (2019). Who is included in the Mad Studies Project? *The Journal of Ethics in Mental Health, 10*, 1–20.

Slater, J., & Liddiard, K. (2018). Why Disability Studies scholars must challenge transmisogyny and transphobia. *Canadian Journal of Disability Studies, 7*(2), 83–93.

Smith, A. (2010). Queer theory and Native Studies: The heteronormativity of settler colonialism. *GLQ: A Journal of Lesbian and Gay Studies, 16*(1–2), 41–68. https://doi.org/10.1215/10642684-2009-012

Smith, N., & Stanley, E. A. (2015). *Captive genders: Trans embodiment and the prison industrial complex.* AK Press.

Somerville, S. (2000). *Queering the color line: Race and the invention of homosexuality in American culture.* Duke University Press.

Spade, D. (2006). Mutilating gender. In S. Stryker & S. Whittle (Eds.), *The Transgender Studies reader* (pp. 315–332). Routledge.

Spandler, H. (2017). Mad and Queer Studies, shared visions? *Asylum: An International Magazine for Democratic Psychiatry, 4*(1), 5–6. https://asy lummagazine.org/wp-content/uploads/2018/03/Asylum-24.1-Mad-Studies-part-2.pdf

Spandler, H., & Barker, M. J. (2016). *Mad and Queer Studies: Interconnections and tensions.* Mad Studies Network. Retrieved August 20, 2021, from https://madstudies2014.wordpress.com/2016/07/01/mad-and-queer-studies-interconnections-and-tensions

Spandler, H., & Carr, S. (2021). A history of lesbian politics and the psy professions. *Feminism & Psychology, 31*(1), 119–139.

Stanley, E. A., & Spade, D. (2012). Queering prison abolition, now? *American Quarterly, 64*(1), 115–127. http://againstequality.org/files/queering_prison_abolition_now.pdf

Stein, M. (2012). *Rethinking the gay and lesbian movement.* Routledge. https://doi.org/10.4324/9780203122211

Stryker, S. (2004). Transgender Studies: Queer theory's evil twin. *GLQ: A Journal of Lesbian and Gay Studies, 10*(2), 212–215. https://muse.jhu.edu/article/54599/pdf

Tam, L. (2013). Whither indigenizing the Mad movement? Theorizing the social relations of race and Madness through conviviality. In B. A. LeFrançois, R. Menzies, & G. Reaume (Eds.), *Mad matters: A critical reader in Canadian Mad Studies* (pp. 281–297). Canadian Scholars Press.

Tosh, J. (2011). "Zuck off!" A commentary on the protest against Ken Zucker and his "treatment" of childhood gender identity disorder. *Psychology of Women Section Review, 13*(1), 10–16.

Tosh, J. (2015). *Perverse psychology: The pathologization of sexual violence and transgenderism.* Routledge. https://doi.org/10.4324/9781315758190

Tosh, J. (2016). *Psychology and gender dysphoria: Feminist and transgender perspectives.* Routledge. https://doi.org/10.4324/9781315794938

Vermette, L. (1988). The 33 years of the lost Indian walk. In B. Burstow & D. Weitz (Eds.), *Shrink resistant: The struggle against psychiatry in Canada* (pp. 117–120). New Star Books.

Vitulli, E. W. (2013). Queering the carceral: Intersecting Queer/Trans Studies and Critical Prison Studies. *GLQ: A Journal of Gay and Lesbian Studies, 19*(1), 111–123.

Waldram, J. (2004). *Revenge of the Windigo: The construction of the mind and mental health of North American Aboriginal peoples.* University of Toronto Press. https://doi.org/10.3138/9781442683815

Walker, N. (2015). *Neuroqueer: An introduction.* Neuroqueer: The writings of Dr. Nick Walker. Retrieved August 20, 2021, from https://neurocosmopolit anism.com/neuroqueer-an-introduction/

Weeks, J. (1985). *Sexuality and its discontents: Meanings, myths and modern sexualities.* Routledge.

Winters, K. (2008). *Gender madness in American psychiatry: Essays from the struggle for dignity.* GID Reform Advocates.

Yellow Bird, P. (2004). *Wild Indians: Native perspectives on the Hiawatha asylum for insane Indians.* Retrieved August 20, 2021, from https://power2u.org/ wp-content/uploads/2017/01/NativePerspectivesPeminaYellowBird.pdf

Zinck, S., & Pignatiello, A. (2015). *External review of the gender identity clinic of the child, youth and family services in the underserved populations program at the centre for addiction and mental health.* TransAdvocate.com. Retrieved August 20, 2021, from https://www.transadvocate.com/wp-con tent/uploads/GIC-Review-26Nov2015-TA1.pdf

3

Expanding the Struggle Against Queer and Trans Pathologization: Challenging Biomedicalism

In the last chapter I argued that attempts to "rescue" some LGBTQ people from the categorization of madness and the accompanying discrimination associated with being considered mentally ill leaves the biomedical model and all of its attending problems intact. Diagnoses that target sexual and gender dissidence such as homosexuality, gender identity disorder (GID), and gender dysphoria (GD) are not the only ones that affect queer and trans people, and some of the critiques of specific diagnoses can in fact further alienate LGBTQ people who experience mental distress. In this chapter I show that advancing a broad critique of the biomedical model while paying attention to the ways in which it specifically affects LGBTQ people provides a more comprehensive understanding of the issues facing LGBTQ people who experience mental distress. I draw on interviews with 37 LGBTQ people who experienced mental distress about their identifications with, and rejections of, various terms, identities, and psychiatric diagnoses. However, this chapter is not simply a discussion of the different ways in which participants self-identified. The participants' rationales for rejecting or embracing various terminologies often point to some of the fundamental problems with the biomedical model itself and indicate the value of a

© The Author(s), under exclusive license to Springer Nature Switzerland AG 2022
M. D. Pilling, *Queer and Trans Madness*,
https://doi.org/10.1007/978-3-030-90413-5_3

mad-queer-trans lens. I apply insights from Mad Studies such as challenging mind/body and mad/sane binaries, resisting the pathologization of marginalized groups, and questioning diagnostic categorizing as a way of making sense of distress. The chapter concludes with a discussion of participants' narratives that located distress in the context of structural oppression and life experiences. The purpose of this chapter is to understand experiences of madness by locating them within social contexts, rather than attributing them to individualized pathologies. This is particularly salient for LGBTQ people, who as members of marginalized groups, experience distress related to homophobia, transphobia, racism, and other forms of oppression. This chapter is, therefore, simultaneously a critique of the biomedical model of mental illness and an argument for the use of a mad-queer-trans lens to make sense of LGBTQ experiences of mental distress. While the main purpose is to critique the biomedical model, it should be noted that a mad-queer-trans lens is also distinct from mainstream LGBTQ mental health research. As discussed in Chapter 1, the mainstream approach acknowledges social context in that it positions LGBTQ people as vulnerable to mental disorders due to homophobia and transphobia. However, this does not challenge the basis of the biomedical model, which locates distress in dysfunctional biological processes. A mad-queer-trans lens demonstrates that mental distress does not have to be biological to be real.

Making Oneself Intelligible: The Importance of Language

Discussions about mental distress are overdetermined by biomedical frameworks and discourses. This speaks to the success of the biomedical model in pervading and dominating both academic and mainstream consciousness. It also indicates the importance of language in structuring frameworks of intelligibility. Many Mad Studies scholars underscore the importance of language in challenging the biomedical model of mental illness (Beresford, 2019; Boyle, 2011; Burstow, 2013). As Boyle (2011) writes, "linguistic devices" are crucial in foregrounding social context, and it would be difficult to do this "without entirely abandoning medical language, including the term 'mental health,' because using this language is the quickest and most effective way of implying lack of intelligibility and suggesting a pathological or deficient individual" (p. 41). Boyle is referring here to mental health practitioners and researchers and acknowledges that jettisoning medical language will be a difficult task given the predominance of "context-free and context-lite language" (p. 41). It is perhaps even more difficult for those who are medicalized and at a power disadvantage to insist on an alternative language. Yet many participants indicated resistance to biomedical terminology and perspectives. It is, therefore, important to explore the implications and possibilities that arise when biomedical model language is challenged or rejected. This challenge is not simply a matter of semantics; it is also about changing the underlying biomedical paradigm. As Beresford (2002) argues, "the interest of mental health service users/survivors in exploring different conceptual frameworks and approaches has become visible through their development of a different language, which replaces the idea of 'mental illness' with terms like 'madness' and 'mental distress'" (p. 582).

The ways in which participants discussed these matters indicate that language use and identity formation are complex and sometimes contradictory. For example, even those who spoke about rejecting medicalized ways of understanding themselves often used diagnostic categories to make parts of their experience intelligible. Again, this exemplifies the difficulty of talking about mental distress in a way that is not medicalized. In some cases, this was due to the permeation of diagnostic terms into colloquial language, such as "depression" and "anxiety." Diagnostic categories also provided a shorthand way of making sense of sets of experiences, thoughts, or behaviours that did not have other readily available names, even when participants questioned the legitimacy of such categorizations. This is indicative of the ways in which ideologies that can be theorized as discrete are not necessarily experienced as such in everyday life. For the sake of coherency, I, therefore, very loosely refer to participants as those who make use of medicalized frameworks to understand themselves and those who challenge such perspectives, based on whether or not this was mostly the case. However, most participants demonstrated an overlapping mixture of ideologies in their narratives, and it is important to note that their perspectives and identities were not static but shifted over the course of time. Moreover, while I expected that there would be strong differences in terms of how participants identified given the presence of mad activist groups in Toronto and the lack of such groups in Winnipeg, this was not the case. I, therefore, do not make distinctions between the Toronto and Winnipeg participants.

Challenging the Mind/Body Dichotomy

Participants who rejected medicalized language often critiqued the biomedical model's approach to understanding the mind as distinct from the body. The mind/body dualism is characteristic of Western medicine and positions mental illness as a phenomenon distinct from physical illness (Porter, 2002). This dualism is normalized as common sense but is in fact a colonial construct. Holistic understandings and practices that do not separate the mind from the body or the person from the environment are part of Indigenous ways of knowing (Stewart, 2008). Some participants critiqued the mind/body dualism. Charlotte,[1] a white, queer, cisgender woman, described the reasons that she did not trust psychiatric approaches to mental illness, based on a critique of this dichotomy:

> We separate brain and body and it's stupid. It makes no frigging sense at all. Because of that I don't trust people because I think that is a big fucking mistake. And it's a lie, also. You can't separate those two things. So having people committed to an entire industry where that's what they do, I'm like, "your entire freaking practice is based on bullshit so how am I really supposed to trust that much of what you have to say?" It's the same problems that I have with the mainstream Western medical model.

For Charlotte, as for other participants, the belief in the mind and body as distinct cast doubt on the veracity of psychiatric ideologies and practices. Similarly, Louise, a white, queer, cisgender woman, said:

> All the aspects of my being are really inter-connected and it's impossible to separate them into one issue or one piece of myself that can

be sick while the others are not or vice versa. So "mentally ill" is problematic for me in that sense, because that implies that there isn't that inter-connection.

Louise did not define herself as mentally ill because it implied that mental and physical health were mutually exclusive. Another participant, Grace, a Korean, queer, gender-fluid woman, explained how this ideology was problematic for making sense of her experiences:

> If your mind is unwell, that can take a toll on your body in lots of ways. Stress can weaken your immune system. But also if you're in a bad emotional mental place, then you can also not take care of your body in the way that you normally would. And that has an impact on your physical health. For me personally I have PTSD [post-traumatic stress disorder] and my seizures are very much a unification of the two because trauma and certain situations and stress trigger a physical manifestation. And I don't really understand how that happens and the doctors don't either. But I see them as together.

Grace explained how her experiences of mental distress were intimately connected to a physical manifestation that took the form of seizures. As Jared, a white, omnisexual trans man, said, the term mentally ill implies that this cannot be the case:

> Oh, mentally ill. Oh, well, I hate that one. Because that just says that some people are healthy and some people are ill and I'm one of the ill people. And mental health is separate from physical health and it's, you know, I have mental problems. Yeah, so that one does not sit well with me. It sounds like something that a doctor would call a patient in a not-helpful way.

Jared succinctly summarized a number of issues with the term mentally ill, including the implied mind/body binary and the power of mental health care professionals to define the experiences of others.

Challenging the Mad/Sane Binary

Jared's comments also challenge the distinction that is generally made between those who are mad and those who are sane. Attempts at understanding mental distress as a part of everyday life experienced by many people challenges one of the fundamental characteristics of the biomedical model: the dichotomous categorizing of people as either sane or mentally ill. A critique of the binary distinction between mad and sane and the pathologizing of the mad that accompanies this dichotomy is common among scholars seeking other ways to conceptualize madness. For example, Bentall (2003) argues that "the 'us' and 'them' distinction has had a number of very serious negative consequences for those living at the mad end of this spectrum," including the suppression of the voices of those deemed mad and harmful medical 'treatments' such as insulin induced comas, electroshock therapy, and leucotomy (p. 496). According to Bentall, the evidence shows that "we are mad to varying degrees, that the boundaries of madness are subject to negotiation, and that some of us get on very well despite being (in psychiatric terms) quite psychotic for much of the time" (p. 496).

Many of the participants reflected this view in their explanations of why they did not identify with the term mentally ill. For example, Daxton, a white, French Canadian, queer, gay, cisgender man, depathologized his experiences of depression and anxiety, stating that he did not describe himself as mentally ill because he thought of his mental health as "not being perfect but as par for the course" because "a lot of people deal with depression, whether it's acute or temporary or long-term." Another participant, Kylie, a white, queer, genderqueer person, told me that she did not use the terms mentally ill and mad because

> while there might be things that I deal with on a daily basis, they don't define me. And I don't see them as ruling my life. I like to look at it as something like, "okay I'm dealing with this," basically. So that's why I would probably choose to go for "psychiatric service consumer."

Owen, a Black, gay, cisgender man, also saw mad and mentally ill as pathologizing terms that reinforced the mad/sane dichotomy. He did not identify with mad "because of the historical connotations." He elaborated:

> It seems like a word to describe violent, angry, uncontrollable people, which is really marginalizing. If you have psychological issues to call someone "mad" or label them "mentally ill" I feel like it isolates them. And it's something that they need to be quarantined and dealt with for. So I'm not sure if I agree with the use of those words.

Owen pointed to the way in which labelling someone based on a binary understanding was dehumanizing and marginalizing. He, therefore, did not take on any identity-based terms regarding mental distress and simply described his "mental health" as "ambivalent at best." Kylie's and Owen's comments also indicate that the term mad was not always seen by the participants as a non-medicalized term and was sometimes interpreted as akin to mentally ill, perhaps because they had not been exposed to the reclamation of this term.

Resisting the Pathologization of Marginalized Groups

Those who refused to take on the label mentally ill often did so on the basis of resisting the pathologization of marginalized groups. For example, Chase, a white, gay, cisgender man, pointed to how medicalized language could be used to label the behaviour of marginalized people:

> I am averse to using "mentally ill" as a descriptor. Especially because it's so ambiguous. You know, I use the example of a woman who's homeless on the street begging for money...kind of mumbling to herself and rocking back and forth and not making eye contact with anyone. And then you have down the street a man coming, dressed sharp...who steps over her...looks at her, scoffs "get a job" and continues to walk away. Who is mentally ill? It's such a weird term that someone who shows signs of "mental health problems," and then you have someone who can be so cruel when they have the means to offer maybe an iota of support.

Chase rejected the label mentally ill because it was often applied to those who engaged in behaviour that was perceived to be socially undesirable or morally reprehensible, which, as Chase's comments indicate, is a subjective judgment based on social values that tend to target the marginalized. He, therefore, did not refer to himself with medicalized terms and chose to call himself a "mad man with a box." Chase described having the freedom to challenge medicalized language and created alternatives as part of his privilege as a young white man living in the Global North:

> I'm a twenty-year old white male living in North America, I'm the least oppressed person on the continent, so it kind of plays to my benefit to challenge stereotypes and archetypes. And it's almost my duty, it's all of our duty if we're able, to rise up and fight oppression systematically and institutionally.

As Chase's comments indicate, part of the reason he was able to resist labels such as mentally ill was due to his white male privilege.

Racialized participants had a heightened awareness of the negative effects of the pathologizing of Black, Indigenous, and people of colour (BIPOC) based on their experiences of racism. For example, Ameena, a South Asian, queer, cisgender woman, explained that as a teenager, she had avoided being psychiatrized at all costs. She had experienced the many "stereotypes of brown people and brown fathers especially" that characterize "young brown girls" as "victims of this patriarch." Ameena was asked by counsellors to "validate this narrative" and feared that her behaviours would be categorized as symptomatic of mental illness and would validate racist stereotypes about her family. As she said,

> It would have torn into my family. It would have made it very difficult for us to continue the way that we were....To feed into this idea of this patriarchal brown male with young daughters would have been really hard. That's why I wouldn't talk about any of these things and I was aware enough to hide the things that I was doing.

Ameena's experiences point to the problematic pathologizing of racialized people that is characteristic of the biomedical model, and she rejected medicalized terms. In response to my questions as to why, she responded:

Well [laughs] because they're fucked up. Why do I reject them? Because they are socially constructed and they are used to disciple people and regulate people and especially people who are located in certain spaces or have other experiences of oppression as well. So it's pathologization of certain behaviours used to govern people. That's why I feel I can't accept that language.

Ameena drew attention to the ways in which medicalized terms are not "just words" but reflect underlying ideologies that are used as tools of social control, targeting people of colour in particular. She was successful in avoiding the psychiatric system and the forceful application of labels such as mentally ill. For this reason, she also did not use any reclamatory terms like "psychiatric survivor" or indeed, as she put it, "any identity-based categories related to mental health or madness." Instead, she stated, "I guess the closest I would come would just be to say that I relate to madness without necessarily taking it on."

Trans participants had also experienced the effects of pathologization and were, therefore, often critical of the biomedical model and its terminology. For example, Jonah, a white, bisexual, trans man, said:

"Mentally ill," I don't know if I've ever actually considered that as something that I would use to describe myself....I don't ever really want to define myself as "ill." That's just another way to pathologize myself in a way that doesn't feel comfy and fun like "crazy" sometimes.

Jonah implicitly suggested that he was already familiar with (and rejected) the negative effects of internalizing pathologization ("just another way to pathologize myself"), perhaps on the basis of sexuality and gender identity. He called himself a psychiatric survivor in order to indicate "the abuses I've had at [the] hand of the system and how I've survived that instead of just kind of pinning myself with a very pathologized idea."

Likewise, Carter, a white, queer, trans man, likened his rejection of the term mentally ill to his rejection of the pathologization of his trans identity. He said that while others labelled him as mentally ill, he did not take on this label:

> Similar to not feeling wrong about being trans, I don't feel ill. You know, I feel like I have hard things that happen in my life, but so does everybody else and so it's a process of trying not to minimize that but also finding what works for me and I am really wary of psychiatric avenues.

Carter managed to avoid psychiatric services for many years and, therefore, also did not take on terms such as psychiatric survivor or psychiatric service user. The term he chose to self-identify was "pervert":

> It's something that's been applied to queer and trans folks for a really long time. And then to add the element of being kinky into that is interesting because I feel like it's really normalized within queer communities, but when I think about it outside of that, most people would consider how I live my life and do my relationships and sex to be really perverted. But I also kind of enjoy that. That's part of being queer for me, is being something that's really unpalatable to heteronormative society. I feel like I gain a lot of power from that label. It feels like part of a big "fuck you" to standards of what relationships and sex should look like.

Carter reclaimed pervert, a term that has its origins in medicine as a way to pathologize non-normative sexualities, genders, desires, and behaviours, and in doing so also resisted the positioning of gender and sexual dissidence as illness.

Making Sense of Mental Distress Through Psychiatric Diagnosis

Many of the participants had mixed feelings about using psychiatric diagnoses to make sense of their experiences. Mad Studies scholars and others who critique the biomedical model have challenged the scientific validity of diagnostic categorizations and claim that the evidence overwhelmingly points to mental distress as an understandable response to structural oppression, trauma, and adverse life experiences (Bentall, 2003; Boyle, 2007; Kinderman et al., 2013; May, 2007; Tew, 2011; Thomas, 2013). Some have pointed to the ever-growing roster of psychiatric diagnoses pathologizing an increasingly large list of behaviours, emotions, and experiences of distress, leading to questions about whether anyone could be deemed mentally healthy (Davis, 1997; Rapley, 2012; Tosh, 2017). Mad Studies scholars have also pointed to the gendered, sexualized, classed, and raced character of psychiatric diagnosis (Fernando, 2010; Joseph, 2014; Metzl, 2009; Terry, 1999; Tosh, 2015, 2016).

However, these discussions often remain at the theoretical level and do not examine how people experience the diagnostic process (May, 2007; Tucker, 2009). As May (2007) argues, the process of receiving a psychiatric diagnosis transforms distress into a medicalized, individualized problem. Being given a diagnosis can have a huge impact on identity and experience. As Tucker (2009) writes, diagnosis is a form of social recognition with many negative associations and has the "power to form identities that exist across multiple contexts…and become the prime identifying feature" (p. 4). Indeed, as one participant, Monica, a white, queer, cisgender woman, said about her diagnosis,

> I find that it's a huge part of my identity....I often feel like that's a bigger part of my identity than my gay identity. I feel like that one, it comes first....It's kind of my top layer of identity, I guess.

It is, therefore, important to examine how the participants negotiated the diagnostic process, as it reveals much about both the appeal of, and the problems with, the biomedical model as it is experienced. Psychiatric diagnoses are the predominant way of explaining experiences of madness, but the participants' narratives reveal that there are many problems with this method of making sense of mental distress.

Some scholars suggest that the limited value of a psychiatric diagnosis to those who receive one is in finding an explanation for their distress (Boyle, 2007; Kinderman et al., 2013; Tucker, 2009). As Kinderman et al. (2013) state,

> while some people find a name or a diagnostic label helpful, our contention is that this helpfulness results from a knowledge that their problems are recognized (in both senses of the word), understood, validated, explained (and explicable) and have some relief. (pp. 2–3)

The participants' narratives supported this contention. For some participants, being given a diagnosis offered relief in that they finally had a way to interpret behaviours, feelings, and thoughts that were frightening and problematic. As Gia, a white, gay, cisgender woman, said about her diagnosis:

> It helps explain a lot of my behaviours, too. So it's good to finally know that there was something wrong with me when I was [pauses]. Like I can recall having episodes when I was young but never identified or anything like that. So it kind of gives me comfort knowing that at least it's a condition that I do have. But unfortunately there's still a lot of people that really don't understand it.

Gia was able to take comfort in having an explanation for behaviour that had caused her problems throughout her life, even though she struggled with other people's lack of understanding of her experiences. Similarly, Jackie, a white, lesbian, cisgender woman, told me it was "nice to have a definitive knowledge of what's wrong with you."

Ironically, participants often stated that being diagnosed with a mental illness was a relief because it meant that they were "not crazy." This underscores the extent to which crazy has come to signify without reason, irrationality, and unintelligibility. For example, Kelsey, a white, bisexual, queer, cisgender woman, said, "it's kind of like, oh good, so it's something real, it's not just all in my head, it's not because I'm crazy, it's not just me." Similarly, Daxton, a white, French Canadian queer, gay, cisgender man, said it was "a relief" to be diagnosed:

> It had been a while that I was kind of like, "what the hell is going on, why do I feel this way." So it was like, okay, at least I have sort of an answer to what this is and I'm not making it up. I'm not, it's funny [pauses] um, you know I was just about to say, "I'm not crazy." It's like, "Oh I have depression, I'm not crazy" [laughs].

Though a psychiatric diagnosis often means that those diagnosed will be perceived as crazy by many, an explanation sometimes provided relief, even if only temporarily, for some of the participants. Mental health care professionals made sense of participants' behaviours, experiences, and thoughts that had become troublesome and provided an answer to what was problematic for the participants.

The participants also expressed other powerful reasons for accepting biomedical explanations for their experiences. Many demonstrated that they were often encouraged to do so by family members and friends. Jackie, a white, lesbian, cisgender woman, described this as follows:

> I think I've come to accept it now. It's been a long time. A couple of friends that have sat with me as I bawled and fought it and was angry and wanted to move past it, they sat there and said, "No, this is it. You're probably going to have to take medication the rest of your life." You never see that for yourself, but I think there's an acceptance of it now.

Jackie described an initial resistance to her diagnosis, which she came to accept with the help of her friends. Collin, a white, gay, cisgender man, described the impact of hearing his family members explain how they felt and how this explained his own experiences:

> My mom has depression and so does my brother. They are on medication for it and they go see a psychiatrist. I didn't realize until they were describing how they felt and I went, "Oh that's really how I felt for two or three years." And I was like, "Oh well, I guess that was why I felt that way."

Collin's distress started to make sense to him within the framework used by his mother and brother. For many participants, the role of support networks was key in reinforcing diagnostic categorization as the best way to understand their experiences.

Participants who accepted their diagnoses as the truth about their experiences did not discuss aspects of the diagnoses that did not accurately describe them. Some, however, expressed ambivalence about fully redefining their sense of self in accordance with the biomedical model. When I asked Misty, a Black, queer, cisgender woman, about her relationship to her diagnoses, she told me that this was something she was "really trying to understand." She explained this as follows:

There was kind of a stale point where I was diagnosed with depression until now with this new diagnosis and I wasn't on medication and I thought these fluctuations in mood were just my personality. I thought maybe I was just upset, like I just had bad coping skills with school or it was just part of the way that I was and I almost started to value [pauses], I mean I think I do still value, the days that are bad because I feel like they give me my personality. And they're valuable to me because that's what I have to offer. It's difficult for me to let go of it, for example with medication, because I feel like it's become so much a part of who I am. Now I'm trying to understand how my life can be, how I can be me as a person with mental illness versus someone who's trying to realign myself every day.

Misty was in the midst of grappling with a changing sense of self and hesitated to fully accept the medicalization of certain emotions and personality traits. Yet she felt strongly that her moods were more than just "a bad day" or "just stress" and that there was "something wrong" that the biomedical model of mental illness could explain and perhaps fix through psychiatric medication.

The hope that medical explanations could lead to resolving distress was common. As Nova, a Métis, lesbian, cisgender woman, said,

I can't fight this problem if I don't know what the problem is so I have to first of all identify what the issue is and then I can go about trying to fix it. You know, because I can't keep going on the way I'm going.

Nova was hopeful that a diagnosis would lead to answers about how to address her distress. As will be discussed more in the following chapter, treatments based on the biomedical model worked for some participants, providing another reason to accept their diagnoses as valid. Beresford and Wallcraft (1997) point out the biomedical model may be the only framework people encounter to explain how they are feeling, and "the idea of 'mental illness' is internalized…as a result of their broader socialization and passage through the psychiatric system" (p. 70). Indeed, the dominance of the biomedical model can occlude other perspectives. Speed (2011) argues that it does not co-exist well with other ideologies:

> If the service user draws from a medical discourse to explain their situation (invoking a chemical imbalance in the brain, for example, as the reason they have auditory hallucinations) then it becomes very difficult for that same person to blame, for example, poverty or abuse they experienced as a child. (p. 125)

It is also important to note that those who dispute the medicalization of their experiences or the veracity of their diagnosis are seen to be lacking "insight," a term that indicates that a person believes they are sick and accepts a biomedical explanation for their illness (Pilling et al., 2018). Showing a lack of insight is sometimes seen by health care practitioners as "a cardinal feature of psychosis" (Bentall, 2003, p. 496). It can, therefore, be risky to disagree with one's diagnosis, as this is seen as a sign of illness and can lead to further medicalization and coercive treatment. This is especially the case for those who are marginalized by racism, classism, homophobia, and other kinds of oppression (Pilling et al., 2018).

Further, a diagnosis is often required for receiving accommodations in the workplace and at school. This can create a necessity to acquire a diagnosis even if it is not desired or experienced as otherwise unhelpful. A diagnosis, therefore, serves several important functions.

Resisting Diagnosis

However, as the first half of this chapter demonstrates, some participants did not unequivocally accept medicalized explanations for their distress. Many critiqued the diagnostic process and diagnostic categorization as a way of interpreting their experiences. It is, therefore, important to examine how people who experience mental distress come to resist the disciplinary power of diagnosis. This discussion also indicates some of the problems with diagnostic categorization as a way of making sense of mental distress.

Some participants who critiqued the biomedical model discussed developing a critical sensibility in university and applying that lens to their understanding of diagnosis and biomedical frameworks. Trevor, a white, queer, trans man, said he learned to question diagnosis and biomedical ways of thinking about madness "through education," which led him to think of "medical or scientific discourse" as "failures": "So I don't see that as a solution anymore, as much as I would like to." Trevor indicated that he no longer had faith in psychiatry and diagnostic processes in part because of what he had learned in school. Likewise, Jonah, a white, bisexual, trans man, said that "some of the most persuasive things and some of the things that guided me along to becoming comfortable with that term [psychiatric survivor] was really just my relationship with the things that I was reading in the academy." Owen, a Black, gay, cisgender man, explained that the more he learned about the DSM, the more he came to think that it was based on a "process that's rooted in cultural conventions." The result was that "I don't trust diagnosis." Owen shifted his understanding of diagnosis and madness from a biologically essentialist perspective to one that focused on social and cultural factors, through his learning in university:

> It's been a process for me of learning about it because I always thought of myself as fairly, it was either I wasn't very smart or I wasn't very able, or I was just not good enough in terms of biology or mental make-up because I turned out gay. It was a long struggle and then the more I think about things I feel like it's more cultural, so I'm really interested in research into how shame is socially constructed and how violent shame and silencing can be.

Owen pointed to how his learning helped him challenge internalized homophobic ideologies that position queer people as biologically and mentally deficient, which sparked an interest in social factors leading to mental distress.

Similarly, Ameena, a South Asian, queer, cisgender woman, said she was predisposed to critique biomedical explanations of mental distress because she "became a lot more political and a lot more aware of systems and power and oppression" through her experiences of being diagnosed with a physical disability. Ameena had been an undergraduate student at this time and had begun to look more closely at the studies presented in class:

What I started seeing was all these stereotypes built into diagnosing and labeling in the studies that we were reading about. Not everyone read through them in detail but I was the kind of person that would read these things, and methodology especially, and I saw how they were drawing diagnoses for certain things based on surveys of twenty white college students.

When Ameena critiqued the methodology of these studies in her papers on these grounds, she was "met with a lot of resistance" from teaching assistants and professors. This only fed her interest in looking at "what's really happening in terms of labeling and diagnostic process and how much is built on these really ridiculous assumptions and power dynamics."

As Ameena's comments also indicate, psychiatric diagnoses are heavily gendered, sexualized, and racialized. As Metzl (2009) argues, interactions between doctors and patients are in part predetermined by institutional racism:

Race impacts medical communication because racial tensions are structured into clinical interactions long before doctors or patients enter examination rooms. To a remarkable extent, anxieties about racial difference shape diagnostic criteria, health-care policies, medical and popular attitudes about mentally ill persons, the structures of treatment facilities, and ultimately, the conversations that take place there within. (p. xi)

While Metzl is referring specifically to race, his arguments also apply to gender and sexuality. Like Ameena, many of the participants critiqued the diagnostic process based on their critical consciousness about power, race, gender, and sexuality.

For example, Jordan, a Black, lesbian, trans person, told me that she did not trust psychiatric diagnoses because of many disciplinary experiences with systemic power throughout her life. She said that her experiences as a youth with the police and with Child & Family Services (CFS) convinced her that "any sort of person who wore a uniform or had some form of power to be able to control you or apprehend you, you know, sucks." Agents of the state such as police and CFS often act as disciplinary forces in BIPOC communities, and Jordan explained that she saw doctors as yet another vector for institutional power "that will tell you what they think is right." Her perspective was also shaped by her experiences in prison, where she was assessed by a psychiatrist and a psychologist:

> It was a part of assessing my rehabilitation or whether I can be released. The psychologist was like, "You're perfectly fine, and you know a lot, and you're pretty smart." And the psychiatrist was like, "You're gonna be a career criminal" [both laugh]. I think that was also because the psychiatrist was working for the prosecutors. I just remember that standing out for me as like, "Okay, you just assigned me the rest of my life."

The stark contradiction in the assessments of Jordan demonstrated for her that diagnostic processes were subjective judgments structured by systemic power relations. Though she did not overtly name racism as part of this process, her narrative can be read with this in mind given that anti-Black racism operates on a systemic level (Maynard, 2017).

Some participants drew attention to the gendered character of diagnostic categorization. Kylie, who identified as a white, queer, genderqueer person, described seeing a psychiatrist who diagnosed her with three mental disorders. She was critical of one in particular, because of her knowledge about how this diagnosis was gendered:

> That makes zero sense to me. I don't like that label because the label was something that has been used against women many times in the past....In terms of my gender identity, sometimes I identify more female and sometimes I'm more male. But sometimes I don't feel like I'm either. But biologically I'm female. So this diagnosis is something that a lot of women get slapped with and it kind of made me go, "If I was a guy would you be saying this to me right now?" And I'm sitting there and I'm going, "This is absurd."

Kylie resisted the diagnosis because her experience as genderqueer and her knowledge about the gendered nature of the diagnosis meant that it did not make sense as a way to describe her experiences. Likewise, Trevor, a white, queer, trans man, recognized the gendered, racialized, and classed nature of psychiatric diagnoses and, therefore, resisted the diagnosis he had been given as a teenager:

> Being white and middle class and a young teenage girl, for sure. Of course you're depressed. Of course you need to be on anti-depressants [laughs]. Like his [the doctor's] attitude was just that probably most teenage girls should be on anti-depressants. So that was another factor in thinking that maybe it wasn't the right thing, that it was kind of a blanket prescription and everybody was going to be getting it who walked into that office.

Trevor's critical consciousness about sexism and medical practice allowed him to critique the diagnostic process and resist the medicalization of his experiences of distress.

Many of the trans participants had an especially fraught relationship with diagnostic processes and categorization. Many had been diagnosed with GID[2] in addition to various other mental disorders. Unlike most of the diagnoses in the DSM, the gendered nature of GID is explicit, making it easy to critique. The veracity of GID is widely questioned within trans scholarship and communities and many do not accept the pathologization of gender nonconformance. Knowledge circulates among trans people about the narrative that must be performed about their experiences, thoughts, and behaviours in order to receive a diagnosis, which is often needed to access the technologies of medical transition.[3] Many trans people, therefore, have a sense of GID as socially constructed, which gives them a level of agency about the diagnostic process in that many recognize the necessity of using the psychiatric system and the diagnosis of GID in a pragmatic way. As Robin, a white, queer, transgender person, said,

> I think it's a bit of a crap issue, honestly [both laugh], and I bit the bullet to jump through the hoops to get the testosterone, so I didn't really dispute their terms very much. I tried to frame my own experience in my own terms but not deviating super far from what they understand as gender identity disorder.

While many trans participants expressed an ability to use GID strategically, going through the diagnostic process also had an impact on their self-understanding. For example, Jared, a white, omnisexual trans man, discussed the complex effects on his sense of self as a result of "re-narrating" his life to fit the diagnostic criteria of GID. Before seeking the diagnosis, Jared was "pretty strongly feminist" in that he was "against gender" because he believed that "a lot of gender had to do with patriarchy." Jared found that his feminist belief that gender was a "social system about power relations" was incompatible with the individualization of diagnostic criteria. While Jared remained critical of the biomedical model, his experiences with the diagnostic process shifted his feminist beliefs:

> Re-narrating my life, re-narrating everything that I thought was politically and socially important into just a sense of who I am as a person and how I fit in the world, was difficult because it involved accepting some dominant ideas about gender and also recognizing that some things were true, that not everybody, actually, was driven by this serious obsession and upset-ness about gender; a lot of people are just fine with it. So that was kind of hard for me, because the politicized view that I had enabled me to not actually address my own situation. So it was a combination of letting go of some of my politics, really, but also incorporating myself more into how I see the world and how I am in the world. So it was tricky.

Jared began the diagnostic process with a strong critique of GID and the biomedical model, but his experiences with diagnosis caused him to conclude that some parts of feminist ideology were incompatible with the realities of trans experience. This had a profound impact on his politics and his sense of self.

As the participants' narratives demonstrate, there are a number of factors influencing their perceptions of the biomedical model of mental illness. These include the relief of finding a way to explain their experiences, connections with family and friends, exposure to alternative frameworks in university and community settings, and applying critical understandings of race, gender, and sexuality to the biomedical model of mental illness.

As discussed at the beginning of this chapter, the biomedical model of mental illness is so prevalent that it was difficult for the participants to make their experiences intelligible without using the language of diagnosis, even when they did not fully agree with diagnosis as an organizing framework for their experiences. If diagnosis is an inadequate way of making sense of experiences of distress, how can these experiences be described?

Some scholars argue that it is helpful to shift from a language of symptoms and diagnoses to that of complaints. Following Bentall (2003), Tew (2011) argues that the language of illness should be replaced by descriptions of "the specific experience that is troubling us," such as hearing voices or persistent distressing thoughts (Tew, 2011, p. 29). For Boyle (2011), this kind of descriptive language should also foreground the context in which the complaints arise. She gives an example to illustrate her point: "The critical voices John hears may be part of a painful debate he is having with himself about whether he cared enough for his wife when she was dying" rather than the terse, medicalized "John is a widower with psychotic symptoms" (p. 41). Bentall (2003) argues that using this kind of descriptive language rather than medicalized terminology dispenses with the need to create a definitive distinction between madness and sanity or to always assume that certain experiences are pathological (p. 141).

Some participants who rejected the term mentally ill were sometimes at a loss for language that felt comfortable and accurately described their experiences. Some found it more helpful to name their specific struggles rather than taking on the pathologizing identity of mentally ill. As Kelsey, a white, bisexual, queer, cisgender woman, said,

> I don't know if it's because of the word illness. I'd rather say that I've struggled with depression. And I struggled with, you know, suicidal thoughts, tendencies too. I mean I could admit that I have an illness with my other recovery programs but maybe it's just like I said, the word "illness" kinda throws me off.

Similarly, Daxton, a white, French Canadian, queer, gay, cisgender man, described himself as someone who experienced feelings of depression and who had "dealt with suicidal tendencies." The linguistic strategies used by participants reinserted the social context that is often stripped by individualizing diagnostic labelling of people's experiences. The next section will further clarify the kinds of experiences that are crucial in providing a social context for understanding mental distress.

A Mad-Queer-Trans Lens: Resisting Individualization and Understanding Social Context

The biomedical model and prevailing assumptions dictate that in order for various social phenomena to be "real," they must be based in biology (e.g., genes, chemical imbalances) despite the fact that many of the social constructs (e.g., time and money) that dictate our lives are clearly real in that they have significant material consequences. Queer Studies scholars have shown that sexuality and gender are real and yet they are not based in biology, that is, there is no gay gene nor is there a biologically based male/female binary (Butler, 2004; Fausto-Sterling, 2000). The ways that humans understand sexuality and gender change according to culture and across historical contexts, and it follows that these shifting social constructs are not biological. And yet, sexuality and gender are real, and society is organized around these concepts in such a way as to have material consequences. Likewise, distress does not have to be caused by biological factors to be real. As Tosh (2016) argues, the biomedical model often results in assumptions that "for someone's suffering to be considered 'real', it needs to have a biological basis. Those who research violence and abuse know this to be untrue" (p. 4).

Many participants drew attention to the ways in which structural oppression and their life experiences played a role in their mental distress. This was in direct contradistinction to the biomedical model, which individualizes distress, attributing the cause to biologically based pathologies, such as chemical imbalances in the brain, rather than taking into account the structural conditions and life experiences that can lead to distress and behaviours that get categorized as non-normative and symptomatic of mental illness. As Rapley et al. (2011) write, ignoring the social context means that "more or less understandable reactions to life's challenges" get turned "into internal individual pathology—whether labeled as depression, psychosis or some other diagnosis" (p. 4). It also means that structural oppression is minimized or ignored. As Ballou and Brown (2002) argue, the individualization characteristic of the biomedical model both silences those deemed mad and fails to take into account "forces, dynamics, and structures" that may lead to experiences of madness. As they state, "while individual problems are certainly significant, it is also significant and meaningful that individuals are enormously impacted by multiple forces and systems" (p. xviii).

This is particularly relevant to LGBTQ people because of the impact of homophobia, transphobia, racism, and other forms of oppression. As Charlotte, a white, queer, cisgender woman, said,

> I think being who I am and having queer people in my life and being queer myself and sort of living apart from a larger segment of the population, I see people get shit on all the fricking damn time because we're queer or because we're poor or different. The world doesn't always change for us or is not set up for the people that I care about....The queer identity that I have and that the people that I care about have, that prevents them from being able to get what they need from systems that are supposed to support them, informs how I feel crazy sometimes. It's also helplessness a little bit, too. That feeling of helplessness impacts the way that I feel crazy. You know, like that crazy feeling of not being able to do anything, being completely unable to move anything or switch something so it works for people, that gives me anxiety. I think it *should* give me anxiety. I actually think it should give *everybody else* anxiety, to be honest. Like I don't think I should have to have all that. Some fucker should carry that shit for me. Whatever. That's the way it is.

Charlotte directly linked her feelings of "craziness" and anxiety to being queer in a homophobic, oppressive society. From a biomedical perspective, Charlotte's distress and anxiety would be perceived as symptoms of illness characteristic of a disordered mind. Her explanation of her experiences challenged this perspective; her anxiety response made sense within the social context she provided. As Boyle (2011) argues, the biomedical model renders experiences of madness unintelligible through sidelining the social context in which these experiences arise. This supposed lack of intelligibility of behaviours and thoughts deemed mad is often what justifies the use of the biomedical model "or any model based on individual deficits" (p. 40). It is, therefore, crucial to insist on the intelligibility of mental distress and behaviours and thoughts that seem abnormal through focusing on "the idea that people's feelings and actions are consonant with their past and present experiences" and recognizing that "some 'normal' social practices, such as gender role socialization or consumerism" can in fact be deeply injurious (p. 41).

It is clear that experiences of oppression based on gender and sexual dissidence are linked to mental distress. For example, Levi, a white, Jewish, gay, cisgender man, described the oppressive treatment of boys and men who transgressed the norms of masculinity and the ways in which this could lead to mental distress:

> I was queer from the very get go. What I liked, what I wanted was totally against the gender role that I was supposed to have. What was great about it is [that] I was bold enough and my family was either ignorant enough or lenient enough that I went and did what I wanted to do and avoided those things I wasn't interested in....The intersection of that with what I would call mental illness is the degree of harassment I experienced all the way through my childhood and my teenage years and in my twenties from my society....I believe that the distress that was constantly on me, the world's response to my being, is a powerful wounding element. And I think there's no way of knowing what would have happened had my orientation and identity not been responded to in the way that it was, with acts of omission of people who did not come to my rescue, or did not come to protect me, or change the situation....I think how they intersect, then, is my identity, the world's response, and then the condition that developed in me because of that intersection.

While Levi valued the experiences created by being able to embrace his queer gender, he identified society's response to it as part of what led to what he called his mental illness. Similarly, Dustin, a white, queer, gay, cisgender man, described the impact of being expected to embody hegemonic masculinity:

This is going back to my experiences with bullying and my own insecurities with not wanting to kiss girls in elementary school or [wanting to] be in art club or all of those kinds of things that made it possible for youth to pick on me were ways in which I deviated from proper pieces of masculinity. And so because I was feminized in the things that I liked...I think I internalized a lot of that. Especially when it came to my body image. And I think body image has a lot to do with how I understand myself to be very insecure. But then how that insecurity transposes onto an anxiety disorder. So having an anxiety disorder is my own discomfort with myself. So being called fat all the time when I was younger. And now seeing myself as someone who is fat, even though I'm not a fat person, but I can't get that out of my head. Or never having a partner...until I was in my fourth year of university because I was so scared of how people would see my body, understand myself as a queer person or a gay person. And I think that has a lot to do with how I became a problem to the psychiatrist. But I also think that my own self-worth was compromised because of all that bullying and sexual assault that I experienced.

Dustin drew attention to the negative impact of being harassed as a child for not living up to the norms of hegemonic masculinity. He explained how this harassment and the effects of fatphobia, homophobia, and sexual assault were directly related to his experiences of anxiety as well as his psychiatrizationw.[4]

Likewise, Silver, a mixed-race, queer, cisgender person described the importance of many social factors in leading to mental distress, including "homophobia and transphobia and being the target of it and being stigmatized, being able to find a job, being rejected by your family or even milder things." Julie, a white, pansexual, cisgender woman, told me that she was "concerned that regular behaviours are seen in a pathological sense," and the reason for her distress "is because of social factors and situational factors." She went on to say: "I don't think it's something that's wrong with my brain. I think it's something that's wrong with the context in which I grew up." Referring to "the potential trauma that comes with hiding your sexuality in a repressive, potentially conservative environment in which you grow up," she said "that can have an effect on your mental health and your well-being."

In addition to experiencing discrimination, queer and trans people can experience isolation and struggle with finding sources of social support. The distress caused by feelings of isolation, especially at a young age, was a common theme in participant narratives. Collin, a white, gay, cisgender man, described feeling depressed and isolated growing up "in a community where there was one gay kid in our entire school" and feeling "all alone" with no one to talk to while "starting to figure out who I was." Owen, a Black, gay, cisgender man, also described feeling isolated as a teenager:

> Around puberty I felt like I didn't have very many people to talk to. There weren't very many resources in [the country where I lived], so when I tried to look up mental health online, I had a lot of symptoms that corresponded with bipolar disorder. In retrospect it was probably just puberty but I don't know....There was a lot of pressure in terms of still being closeted and being in a very fundamentalist Muslim country. And really my own understanding of that place was fairly limited because I wasn't someone that was enmeshed in that community; I was an immigrant even there. So it felt really isolating. And so that led me to think that I was depressed.

Owen described the impact of isolation in the context of immigration and homophobia, a deeply stressful situation that led to confusion and distress.

Some participants also discussed feeling isolated because of white supremacy and racism. Sean, an East Asian, queer, trans man, discussed the impact of racism and isolation as a person of colour person growing up in a small town:

> I think growing up in [a small town] and not being surrounded by other people of colour, I think that affected my mental health in that I didn't understand what racism really was and so I thought it was just me—that people hated me. It was apparent because you're a "chink" or whatever. I didn't know how to deal with it because there were no classes on it and nothing that reflected my culture in school. And it was also very religious—a Catholic school upbringing. It was hard for me [and my

siblings] who were the only East Asians in our grade for the longest time until we hit high school and there was maybe three more.

Sean described the impact of growing up as a person of colour in a white supremacist society where racism was never named and assimilation was enforced through Eurocentric curricula. His story draws attention to the kinds of practices that are commonly accepted as benign (white-centric curricula) that are in fact harmful and can lead to mental distress.

Trans participants often linked feelings of mental distress to not being able to transition and being forced to live as the gender they were assigned at birth. For example, Kyle, an Indigenous, heterosexual, trans man, described living with extreme levels of distress before gaining access to testosterone:

> I went to see [the doctor] and it was like either I get the sex change or I keep doing drugs until I kill myself. Those are the only two options. I've never been that blunt with a doctor. You know I'm always quiet….I was like either you help with my transition or I just keep on doing drugs till eventually my liver fails or something. Because I'm not a lesbian, I'm sick of living like that, I don't classify myself as a lesbian….So he's helped me out and everything's completely changed. It's like flipping a pancake almost [laughs]. Probably about two months after starting testosterone and even my roommates, my friends noticed. As a youth I'd been in every kind of drug possible, cocaine, heroin, injecting drugs, like I amaze myself that I'm actually still alive, you know [laughs], with some of the stuff I've done….A lot of people have noticed I'm just a lot happier. A lot happier with myself, a lot happier with life and not on a one-way road to destruction.

Kyle directly linked his mental distress to his social situation. He described feeling anxious and depressed for many years until he began transitioning. At that point, his level of mental distress decreased exponentially and he was able to stop taking psychiatric medications. Similarly, Maya, a white, French Canadian, lesbian, transgender woman, told me that she had "life-long depression and transitioning is the cure." She described being diagnosed with depression and trying psychiatric drugs in the hopes that they would help her feel better. After four years of taking various psychiatric medications, she came to the realization that she was trans:

> At that point I started getting worse because it's like I knew what I needed to do to cure myself but I was in a situation where I couldn't pursue that. So the knowledge and not being able to do anything about it made it worse and so we tried to fight that with more medication. What happened was that I attempted suicide. When I stopped myself, clarity came to mind and I said that if I'm going to beat the depression I have to change my gender. At that point I started feeling 100% better. It was at that point I stopped taking medication.

Like Kyle, Maya experienced high levels of mental distress and attempted suicide because of the inability to transition. Once she was able to change her situation and begin transitioning, she noticed a substantial lessening of mental distress and stopped taking psychiatric medications.

Other participants made mention of the impact of traumatic experiences and difficult family relations as something that led to mental distress. Jacy, a Métis, trans, genderqueer person, described experiencing difficulties connected to his mother and her partner overdosing on drugs:

> I was feeling kind of suicidal and self-injured a bit. And I was going through a lot of stuff at that time. I was with my mom. She's a drug user and she O.D.'d when I was eight. And also my mom's partner that she had been with for several years O.D.'d when I was about twelve and was in a coma for a little while and came out of that with brain damage and so I was with him through that, for about a year through that process and seeing him kind of come back to life a bit. Which it's lucky he did. I think it probably brought up a lot of trauma that I had with my mom O.D.-ing.

Jacy's mental distress makes sense when connected with what was going on with his family. As he put it,

> I think it makes sense that I have panic and anxiety. I just have a lot of shit, I guess....I've had a lot of trauma in my life and I think I'm just dealing with that in my body, trying to figure that out.

Similarly, Kelsey, a white, bisexual, queer, cisgender woman, described growing up in an "alcoholic dysfunctional family" and connected her feelings of mental distress to these experiences:

> I'd rather say "survivor" than "mad" or "mentally ill." Like I said, both my parents were alcoholic and well my mom did get into twelve step recovery and she did stop drinking but I feel like she wasn't really what they say, "working her program." She didn't take responsibility. She would act crazy and then act like someone else had the problem.

Kelsey did not see herself as mentally ill because her distress made sense to her given her family dynamics. Likewise, Julie, a white, pansexual, cisgender woman, described her mental distress as the result of her childhood experiences:

> I became homeless at sixteen and I was homeless for two months. I had a very tumultuous upbringing. My parents were very middle class but they were abusive and there was all kinds of emotional abuse that was going on and sometimes physical abuse.

While Jacy's, Kelsey's, and Julie's experiences do not directly speak to the significance of being LGBTQ, it is important to note that the existence of systemic discrimination means that even in cases where structural oppression is not overt, it plays a role. For example, there are high rates of homelessness among LGBTQ people, and being homeless may be that much more difficult as a LGBTQ person because of homophobia, transphobia, and other forms of oppression in homeless shelter systems (Abramovich, 2012; Ecker et al., 2019).

As the participants' narratives demonstrate, considering the role of systemic oppression and life experiences are crucial in understanding mental distress. A mad-queer-trans lens indicates that depathologizing mental distress by locating it within social contexts positions mental distress as an understandable response to structural oppression and life experiences. This is in direct contradistinction to the biomedical model, which frames the mentally ill as unintelligible based on underlying "disorders." As Rimke and Brock (2012) state, the resounding messages provided by the psy complex imply that people's struggles are personal and internally produced, as though our experiences in the world were somehow separate and distinct from the social conditions that shape, produce, and order those experiences. (p. 198)

A mad-queer-trans lens is particularly useful for understanding LGBTQ experiences because marginalized groups contend with homophobia, transphobia, and other forms of oppression. This pushes the queer critique beyond selective diagnoses to make the broader claim that the biomedical model as a whole is problematic and that a mad-queer-trans lens can provide another way of making LGBTQ experiences of madness intelligible. A mad-queer-trans lens also challenges mainstream LGBTQ mental health research that positions queer and trans people as more vulnerable to mental disorder because of discrimination, by demonstrating that mental distress does not have to be caused by biological factors in order to be real. The next two chapters will further demonstrate the importance of a broad critique of biomedicalism by exploring the ways in which medical strategies for addressing distress do not address the systemic issues identified by the participants and can in fact perpetuate them, causing further distress.

Notes

1. All names used are pseudonyms.
2. The interviews took place before gender identity disorder was changed to gender dysphoria in the publication of DSM-5 in 2013.
3. In Canada, the process for medical transition is different in each province. Generally speaking, it is only possible to have surgery without a diagnosis of GID (now GD) if one has the means to pay a private surgeon (and sometimes not even then, as some request evidence of having been diagnosed). This is, therefore, a class stratified situation. It should also be noted that the procedure for gaining access to publicly funded surgery is generally much more invasive and time consuming than private surgery. Those seeking hormones usually also require diagnosis.

4. Fatphobia refers to the pervasive positioning of "thinner bodies as morally, medically, aesthetically, and sexually desirable, while heavy bodes are vilified" as well as the "fear and hatred" directed at "visible body fat on oneself or others" (Saguy & Ward, 2011, p. 54).

References

Abramovich, I. A. (2012). No safe place to go—LGBTQ youth homelessness in Canada: Reviewing the literature. *Canadian Journal of Family and Youth/Le Journal Canadien de Famille et de la Jeunesse, 4*(1), 29–51. https://doi.org/10.29173/cjfy16579

Ballou, M., & Brown, L. S. (Eds.). (2002). *Rethinking mental health and disorder: Feminist perspectives*. Guilford Press.

Bentall, R. P. (2003). *Madness explained: Psychosis and human nature*. Penguin Books. https://doi.org/10.1192/bjp.184.4.374-a

Beresford, P. (2002). Thinking about 'mental health': Towards a social model. *Journal of Mental Health, 11*(6), 581–584.

Beresford, P. (2019). Including our self in struggle: Challenging the neo-liberal psycho-system's subversion of us, our ideas and action. *Canadian Journal of Disability Studies, 8*(4), 31–59.

Beresford, P., & Wallcraft, J. (1997). Psychiatric system survivors and emancipatory research: Issues, overlaps and differences. In C. Barnes & G. Mercer (Eds.), *Doing disability research* (pp. 66–87). Disability Press. http://citeseerx.ist.psu.edu/viewdoc/download;jsessionid=683F451F27347DB6B86C512031CC2AFB?doi=10.1.1.366.2482&rep=rep1&type=pdf

Boyle, M. (2007). The problem with diagnosis. *Psychologist, 20*(5), 290–295. https://thepsychologist.bps.org.uk/volume-20/edition-5/diagnosis-special-issue-part-1-2

Boyle, M. (2011). Making the world go away, and how psychology and psychiatry benefit. In M. Rapley, J. Moncrieff, & J. Dillon (Eds.), *De-medicalizing misery: Psychiatry, psychology and the human condition* (pp. 27–44). Palgrave Macmillan. https://doi.org/10.1057/9780230342507.0007

Burstow, B. (2013). A rose by any other name: Naming and the battle against psychiatry. In B. LeFrançois, R. Menzies, & G. Reaume (Eds.), *Mad matters:*

A critical reader in Canadian mad studies (pp. 79–90). Canadian Scholars Press.

Butler, J. (2004). Undoing gender. *Routledge.* https://doi.org/10.4324/978020 3499627

Davis, L. J. (1997, February). The encyclopedia of insanity: A psychiatric handbook lists a madness for everyone. *Harper's Magazine.* Retrieved August 21, 2021, from https://harpers.org/archive/1997/02/the-encyclopedia-of-ins anity/

Ecker, J., Aubry, T., & Sylvestre, J. (2019). A review of the literature on LGBTQ adults who experience homelessness. *Journal of Homosexuality, 66*(3), 297–323. https://doi.org/:%2010.1080/00918369.2017.1413277.

Fausto-Sterling, A. (2000). *Sexing the body: Gender politics and the construction of sexuality.* Basic Books. https://doi.org/10.1017/S0730938400005232

Fernando, S. (2010). *Mental health, race and culture.* Palgrave Macmillan. https://doi.org/10.1007/978-1-137-01368-2

Joseph, A. J. (2014). A prescription for violence: The legacy of colonization in contemporary forensic mental health and the production of difference. *Critical Criminology, 22*(2), 273–292. https://doi.org/10.1007/s10612-013-9208-1

Kinderman, P., Read, J., Moncrieff, J., & Bentall, R. P. (2013). Drop the language of disorder. *Evidence Based Mental Health, 16*(2–3). https://doi.org/10.1136/eb-2012-100987

May, R. (2007). Working outside the diagnostic frame. *Psychologist, 20*(5), 300–301. https://thepsychologist.bps.org.uk/volume-20/edition-5/diagnosis-special-issue-part-5

Maynard, R. (2017). *Policing Black lives: State violence in Canada from slavery to the present.* Fernwood Publishing.

Metzl, J. (2009). *The protest psychosis: How schizophrenia became a Black disease.* Beacon Press. https://doi.org/10.18061/dsq.v32i1.3021

Pilling, M. D., Daley, A., Gibson, M. F., Ross, L. E., & Zaheer, J. (2018). Assessing "insight," determining agency and autonomy: Implicating social identities. In J. Kilty & E. Dej (Eds.), *Containing madness: Gender and "psy" in institutional contexts* (pp. 191–213). Palgrave Macmillan. https://doi.org/10.1007/978-3-319-89749-3_9

Porter, R. (2002). *Madness: A brief history.* Oxford University Press. https://doi.org/10.1017/s0790966700007060

Rapley, M. (2012). W(h)ither DSM? *Mauritas, 73*(2), 81–82. https://doi.org/10.1016/j.maturitas.2012.06.003

Rapley, M., Moncrieff, J., & Dillon, J. (2011). Carving nature at its joints? DSM and the medicalization of everyday life. In M. Rapley, J. Moncrieff, & J. Dillon (Eds.), *De-medicalizing misery: Psychiatry, psychology and the human condition* (pp. 1–10). Palgrave Macmillan. https://doi.org/10.1057/978023 0342507_1

Rimke, H., & Brock, D. (2012). The culture of therapy: Psychocentrism in everyday life. In M. Thomas, R. Raby, & D. Brock (Eds.), *Power and everyday practices* (pp. 182–202). Nelson.

Saguy, A. C., & Ward, A. (2011). Coming out as fat: Rethinking stigma. *Social Psychology Quarterly, 74*(1), 53–75. https://doi.org/10.1177/019027251139 8190

Speed, E. (2011). Discourses of acceptance and resistance: Speaking out about psychiatry. In M. Rapley, J. Moncrieff, & J. Dillon (Eds.), *De-medicalizing misery: Psychiatry, psychology and the human condition* (pp. 123–141). Palgrave Macmillan. https://doi.org/10.1057/9780230342507_10

Stewart, S. (2008). Promoting Indigenous mental health: Cultural perspectives on healing from native counsellors in Canada. *International Journal of Health Promotion and Education, 46*(2), 49–56. Retrieved August 21, 2021, from https://campusmentalhealth.ca/wp-content/uploads/2018/03/Promoting-Indigenous-Mental-Health-Stewart.pdf

Terry, J. (1999). *An American obsession: Science, medicine, and homosexuality in modern society*. University of Chicago Press. https://doi.org/10.7208/chicago/9780226793689.001.0001

Tew, J. (2011). *Social approaches to mental distress*. Palgrave Macmillan. https://doi.org/10.1080/09687599.2012.722410

Thomas, P. (2013). Pinball wizards and the doomed project of psychiatric diagnosis. In *Mad in America: Science, psychiatry and community*. Retrieved August 21, 2021, from https://www.madinamerica.com/2013/02/pinball-wizards-and-the-doomed-project-of-psychiatric-diagnosis/

Tosh, J. (2015). *Perverse psychology: The pathologization of sexual violence and transgenderism*. Routledge. https://doi.org/10.4324/9781315758190

Tosh, J. (2016). *Psychology and gender dysphoria: Feminist and transgender perspectives*. Routledge. https://doi.org/10.4324/9781315794938

Tosh, J. (2017). Gender non-conformity or psychiatric non-compliance? How organized non-compliance can offer a future without psychiatry. In M. Morrow & L. H. Malcoe (Eds.), *Critical inquiries for social justice in mental health* (pp. 255–282). University of Toronto Press. https://psycnet.apa.org/record/2018-10501-009

Tucker, I. (2009). "This is for life": A discursive analysis of the dilemmas of constructing diagnostic identities. *Forum Qualitative Sozialforschung/Forum: Qualitative Social Research, 10*(3). https://doi.org/10.17169/fqs-10.3.1376

4

The Biomedical Model in Practice I: Encounters with Mental Health Care Practitioners

In this chapter I draw on data from interviews with 37 LGBTQ people who have experienced mental distress to examine their encounters with mental health care practitioners. I explore how the ideologies underpinning mental health care practices govern the relationship between practitioners and those seeking care, as well as decisions about how to address or manage mental distress. I argue that the power relations embedded in the biomedical model make for inequitable relationships and interactions, a problem compounded by a profound lack of knowledge among practitioners about LGBTQ cultures, identities, and ways of being as well as structural racism and colonialism within mental health systems. Furthermore, participants' experiences indicate that despite the removal of homosexuality from the DSM and resistance to the inclusion of gender dysphoria (GD), LGBTQ people continue to be pathologized through various means. These include discourses that position nonnormative sexual and gendered behaviour, desires, and practices as deviant, diagnostic criteria that pathologize "promiscuous" behaviour, and the use of mental health systems and child protective services as tools of colonial violence. My analysis shows that assessments of mental health made by mental health care practitioners whose approaches are informed by

M. D. Pilling, *Queer and Trans Madness*, https://doi.org/10.1007/978-3-030-90413-5_4

biomedicalism are not objective. Rather, they are enculturated processes rife with problematic subjective judgments and discrimination. This demonstrates that structural oppression exists within the mental health system, often resulting in the exacerbation rather than alleviation of distress.

Power Dynamics in Relationships Informed by Biomedicalism

The nature of the relationship between the practitioner and the person experiencing mental distress is crucial, whether the relationship is new or ongoing. Many participants emphasized the importance of trust, collaboration, respect, and allyship and indicated that interactions with practitioners who displayed these characteristics were exceedingly rare in the mental health care system. Mental health practitioners have been positioned as experts, while the knowledge of mental health service users has been disregarded, including their personal experience (Boxall & Beresford, 2013). As discussed in Chapter 3, the biomedical model positions those experiencing mental distress as deficient and in need of correction, as irrational and incapable of making informed decisions, and as fundamentally different from those who are considered sane. These problems are compounded by homophobia, transphobia, racism, and other forms of oppression. While not all individual practitioners explicitly embrace these beliefs, they are implicit in the ideology governing medical practice and informed the way many practitioners interacted with the participants.

A major theme that emerged from the participants' stories about their encounters with practitioners was the unequal power relations that governed these interactions and relationships. Many participants indicated that there was an inherent power imbalance in a model that set up practitioners as all-knowing experts with the power to assess and diagnose those experiencing distress. As Jacy,[1] a Métis, trans, genderqueer person, said:

> I'm generally somebody who can fucking say what I mean and stand up and advocate for myself. But when it comes to doctors and people in health care, there's just such a fucking power dynamic, like power imbalance. There's just nothing you can do.

Participants described interactions that felt cold and distant, with no collaboration and often no respect. Many felt as if practitioners had limited or no regard for their agency. For example, Dustin, a white, queer, gay, cisgender man, described feeling frustrated that his psychiatrist was unwilling to share information with him:

> I met resistance in that counselling work where I really had to ask, "Can I look at my notes?" "No." "Well why? I want to know what you're saying about me. I see you frantically writing, I want to know what you're writing. Are you writing, 'He's really crazy?' Are you writing, 'I'm bored?' Are you drawing a happy face? Like what are you doing?" But they won't share that with you.

Dustin's attempt to equalize the relationship through information sharing was shut down, reducing his trust in his psychiatrist. This lack of transparency was common, with some participants experiencing outright deception from practitioners. Shannon, a white, queer, cisgender woman, described being "tricked into using a psychiatrist" by her general practitioner after telling him that she believed she had fibromyalgia:

> He said he was sending me to a specialist. When I arrived there he started asking me all these questions about my childhood and all that kind of thing and I was like, "Why are you asking me these kind of questions? Are you a rheumatologist or something?" He's like, "No, I'm a psychiatrist. Didn't your doctor tell you that?" And I was like, "Ahh, no."

Shannon needed forms completed by a doctor that would confirm her inability to work in order to receive disability benefits from Manitoba's Employment and Income Assistance program. She believed the psychiatrist had completed these forms based on a diagnosis of fibromyalgia:

He said he would sign my medical forms...but instead of putting fibromyalgia he put borderline [personality disorder] and somatic personality [somatization disorder]. And he hadn't even shared that diagnosis with me. It was shared to me by Employment and Income Assistance.

Shannon was deceived by both her general practitioner and a psychiatrist, who gave her a diagnosis that indicated that he did not believe in the veracity of the fibromyalgia diagnosis and her account of her symptoms.[2] Shannon believed that part of the reason her general practitioner sent her to the psychiatrist was that he saw her as an "insane queer woman." She believed she was seen as less credible by her doctor because he espoused homophobic beliefs and positioned her sexuality as a form of mental illness. As she put it, "Just like, 'You're crazy. Gay.'"

The lack of transparency about diagnosis may be of particular concern for trans people. Trevor, a white, queer, trans man, indicated that he was not told about being given a diagnosis of gender identity disorder (GID), discovering this years later through a third party:

I didn't see the diagnosis until eventually I had a endocrinologist who asked me a lot of psychological questions, which I thought was really weird because she was asking me more personal questions than the shrink actually did. But she eventually gave me all of my health documents when I moved...so I could give it to whatever doctor I'd go in to see. In that I saw some of the original documents and saw that "this patient has been diagnosed with gender identity disorder" on it and realized that I had been subjected to some designations and some pretty specific terms that I didn't realize had been applied to me.

While Trevor was initially surprised, he said, "I guess the assumption is that you know that that's why you're there, so you want to get that designation [both laugh]. I think they would be a little, 'What did you expect?' [laughs]." Trevor was not alone in his unawareness. Other trans participants indicated that they didn't know a diagnosis of GID was required in order to access publicly funded medical technologies of transition. For example, Elias, a racialized, gay, trans man, told me, "I don't think that's how it works out here," despite having already seen the doctor at the trans clinic in Winnipeg. This indicates that there is a lack of clarity and transparency about sharing diagnoses. Though there is a culture of informal knowledge exchange in trans communities, practitioners should not assume that all trans people already know they will be officially diagnosed before being allowed access to medical transition. The importance of this should not be underestimated. Many trans people disagree strongly with the pathologization of trans identities and behaviours and some go to great lengths to avoid having their transition psychiatrized.

Many participants also described condescending and paternalistic practitioners. For example, Kelsey, a white, bisexual, queer, cisgender woman, told me the following about her experience in a hospital in Toronto:

> The questions were just too stupid and we were sitting there for a while and I kind of got annoyed. Like they started asking me, "What day is this?" "What floor are we on?" and "Where are we?" And by that time I felt like saying something smart-ass like "Mars" and, you know, "The forty-first of October." Like shut up. What do you think I'm going to say, right?

It sounds like Kelsey was assessed using a standard tool of psychiatric assessment, the Mental Status Examination. The section she described is aimed at assessing level of cognition but was experienced by her as insulting and paternalistic. As Kelsey's comments suggest, the application of standard assessment may sometimes be at the expense of being attuned and helpful to someone experiencing distress.

Likewise, Grace, a Korean, queer, gender-fluid woman, felt that psychiatrists were not attuned or caring and were instead "formal, not supportive," as well as "offensive, judgmental" and "not really caring about the person." She attributed this to the medical model:

> I think because there's such a medical model with so many psychs that when you're talking about someone's emotional and mental well-being, I feel like you should pay attention to the emotions they're talking about and the mental state that they're in. A lot of the times that doesn't happen. I've had doctors pass comments about the way I look. I recently had a psych tell me that I was defiant. I find it really offensive that the supposed

objective is someone's mental health, but there are insensitive, rude things that are passed [on] that don't even consider where they're at or who they are. Things like my gender and my sexual orientation can often be targeted.

As Grace's story also indicates, the power imbalance between practitioners and those experiencing mental distress is compounded by oppressive beliefs and lack of knowledge about LGBTQ ways of being.

"Going Back to Gender and Sexuality 101": Practitioner Lack of Knowledge About Gender Identity and Sexuality

Participants often came into contact with mental health care practitioners who had little to no knowledge of LGBTQ cultures, identities, ways of being, or the impact of systemic oppression. While this problem is not limited to approaches informed by the biomedical model, medical training generally does little to acknowledge or address this problem (McIntyre et al., 2011; Rutherford et al., 2012). Medical education in Canada and the United States is greatly lacking in attention to LGBT issues (Cooper et al., 2018; Holthouser et al., 2017; Nowaskie, 2020; Obedin-Maliver et al., 2011). Due to its large, diverse population, Toronto may be assumed to be a well-resourced city for LGBTQ people. However, participants in both Toronto and Winnipeg indicated that unless they were receiving services at an LGBTQ organization, they encountered practitioners who demonstrated a profound lack of knowledge about LGBTQ identities, ways of being, and common experiences of oppression.

For example, Julie, a white, pansexual, cisgender woman, described seeing a psychologist in Toronto who could not understand her partnership with a trans woman: "I was like, 'We've spent half these sessions just trying to clarify stuff about transsexuality to you. That's not my job. It's not my job to teach you. You're supposed to be the professional.'" Julie experienced the same problem with a psychotherapist:

She didn't seem to know anything about queer issues or trans issues and any time I talked to her about that stuff it just seemed kind of foreign to her. I don't expect everybody to know everything, but I do expect a degree of something, you know [both laugh]. So that was difficult. I don't want to have to feel like I have to explain the basics, like going back to Gender and Sexuality 101 to set up enough context for my life to make sense to a service provider.

Like Julie, many participants felt like they had to educate service providers about sexuality and gender, making it difficult to focus on the distress they wanted to address and in some cases making it worse. Kelsey, who was assessed at a psychiatric hospital in Toronto, encountered stereotypical thinking about bisexuality:

When I tried to be honest and open, telling them that I was bisexual, then of course they're like, "Well which do you like better?" And I'm just like, making a puking face [both laugh]. You know, "Shut up, who cares, what's it matter, why do I have to choose?" I mean I hate it when people ask me that anyway, but I just felt that was especially insensitive for people in the mental health field.

Kelsey was frustrated with the obvious lack of knowledge about bisexuality and the stereotypes expressed by her practitioners, further reducing her trust in the care provided.

Practitioners who were trans-positive and trans-knowledgeable were particularly hard to find. Jared, a white, omnisexual, trans man, indicated that this was especially difficult to find after transition:

After transition, almost impossible to get anybody who has any kind of understanding of trans issues that are not transition related or that are not gender dysphoria related. So that part I found really hard, because any kind of counselling or any services that I get now, people literally cannot wrap their mind around my history with gender.

For many participants like Jared, this meant that they limited access to health care services. As he said,

I basically can't get services anymore. And that's true for health care, too. In general I'm so far off the map of what's regular that doctors and clinicians are not trained to deal with it....I'm articulate enough that I can say things but they still don't get it.

Though many practitioners had no LGBTQ-specific knowledge, many still behaved like experts in this regard. Jonah, a white, bisexual, trans man, described being seen by a general practitioner:

I get in to the room with the doctor...and he says, "Look, is it possible that you think you're trans but really you're actually bisexual?" And I was like, "Well, I think I've already considered that possibility, and I think that those things don't have anything to do with each other. So no, I think I'm trans *and* bisexual, actually. Uh, you're a jackass." I think that is a really good example of those doctors truly having no fucking clue whatsoever about queer people in general and trans people specifically.

Practitioners like the one seen by Jonah continued to act as if they knew best, despite their glaring lack of awareness. Unsurprisingly, Jonah did not feel as if he could get his health care needs met by this practitioner.

Participants in Winnipeg also reported a widespread lack of knowledge amongst mental health care practitioners. Maya, a white, French Canadian, lesbian, trans woman, told me she felt like she wasted time seeing a psychiatrist who was "a hack" and did not have the knowledge necessary to help her:

I think my psychiatrist has never been trained in GLBT, so I think she didn't have the knowledge and so she was just trying to do whatever she could to make you feel better. But I don't think she knew what she could do to get me through this.

Another Winnipegger, Dana, a white, Portuguese, French Canadian, lesbian, queer person, had the veracity of her lesbian identity questioned by her psychiatrist:

I've talked to her about having sex with guys. And she's like "Are you sure you're a lesbian?"...Nobody had ever questioned that. I was mid-twenties at that point. I think to question that after I'd been out for how many years, it was like, "Yeah I'm a lesbian. I very much don't like sex with guys, although I do it."

Dana's psychiatrist had a rigid understanding of sexual identity categories and was unable to understand that the links between sexual behaviour and identity categories are not always straightforward. This became a sticking point in their sessions, and Dana believed that the psychiatrist continued to see her as someone who was confused and undecided about her sexuality, even though this did not reflect Dana's sense of self.

Encountering practitioners ignorant of LGBTQ identities and ways of being when participants were in a vulnerable position was difficult for many. LGBTQ-specific services have long waiting lists in both Toronto and Winnipeg, making it hard to use these services as an alternative. Additionally, for Black, Indigenous, and people of colour (BIPOC) participants, even LGBTQ-specific services were problematic because of racism.

Racism in Mental Health Care

Queer and trans BIPOC experience intersectional forms of oppression in mental health care services, including within LGBTQ-focused services (Gaspar et al., 2021; Giwa & Greensmith, 2012; Pilling et al., 2017). BIPOC participants experienced heterosexism from practitioners who assumed they were heterosexual, indicating a complex interplay of race-based assumptions and heterosexism. For example, Owen, a Black, gay, cisgender man, told me the following about his encounter with a doctor:

> The doctor asked, "So you have sex with women, right?" and marked off on the paper that I have sex with women and literally asked me three times. He's like, "You have sex with women, right?" I was like "No." And he's like, "No, I mean, do you have sex with women?" And I said, "No." And then it almost sunk in at that point and he was gonna' etch out his mark but before he did that he thought it would be best to say, "No I mean, are you gay?" [both laugh]. I was like, "Yeah." And finally he changed it. For me, that was not so much just homophobic as much as

racist or classist. It's not like I had on my Lady Gaga t-shirt or something. I was wearing what I consider regular clothes, jeans or whatever.

Owen's encounter draws attention to the ways in which heterosexism intertwines with racism and classism to create wealth and whiteness as an integral part of being gay and male in the social imaginary. As a Black, low-income man, he was not read as gay without overtly signifying queerness through white North American norms (e.g., a Lady Gaga t-shirt) and had to actively work against disbelief that he was gay.

Many BIPOC participants also indicated that it was difficult to find service providers who could understand the ways in which racism informed their experiences. As Sean, an East Asian, queer, trans man, said, there is a "lack of awareness" about race and racism among mental health counsellors, including those located in LGBTQ organizations. Sean saw a counsellor at an LGBTQ-focused community centre who "didn't really talk about race that much," though Sean would have liked to. As he put it, "it helps to have that sort of knowledge or people talking about race and understanding like race in general and intersectionalities." When Sean joined an LGBTQ support group about mental distress, he found that when he discussed his experiences of racism, others tried to neutralize the experience as simply bullying. When Sean challenged this, he was made to feel as if he had to "prove that it actually happened."

Another participant, Dylan, a Métis, queer, cisgender man, described being unable to access services because of the "weird idea" that "if you're Aboriginal and you're queer, people don't know what to do with that." He explained, "they either want you to be one or the other. And then if you're in those spaces, it's typically one or the other." This leaves two-spirit and Indigenous LGBTQ people without services that incorporate an understanding of the impact of racism and colonialism on two-spirit or LGBTQ and Indigenous individuals or that pathologize them.

Similarly, Jordan, a Black, lesbian, trans person, saw a counsellor at an LGBTQ-friendly organization in Winnipeg who was unable to relate to her experiences as a Black, genderqueer person. Following her oppressive experience there, Jordan never sought out services again. In fact, when Jordan experienced what she called "a mental breakdown" with "suicidal ideation" in which a mobile crisis unit and the police were involved, she received no support from counsellors. Her cumulative experiences with the mental health care system made her "skeptical and fearful of the whole institution of health care" and she said that she would never be able to "get the services I need." Jordan's experiences can be seen as an example of structural anti-Black racism in the mental health care system, including in LGBTQ service organizations. The result for some, like Logan, a bi-racial, queer, genderqueer person, was to avoid all health care services if at all possible: "Within the past few years, as a very queer unusual person, I've just barred, kept to like the walk-in clinics or just deal with it myself, or [my] grandma." Logan preferred to avoid care or receive care from his grandmother rather than risk oppressive encounters in the mental health care system. As this indicates, mental health care can be a site of oppression for LGBTQ people, especially those who are BIPOC.

Colonialism in Mental Health Care

Two-spirit and Indigenous LGBTQ people have reason to view mental health care practitioners with distrust, as the mental health care system has functioned as a tool of colonization. For example, the system often works in tandem with child protective services in displacing and controlling Indigenous people. Indigenous people have long been deemed mentally ill and institutionalized for resisting colonization (Kanani, 2011; Menzies & Palys, 2006; Vermette, 1988; Yellow Bird, 2004). Moreover, the child protection system in Canada is governed by federal and provincial legislation that does not recognize tribal authority and fails to meet the needs of Indigenous youth, who continue to be over-represented in the system (Baskin, 2007; Bennett et al., 2005). As de Leeuw et al. (2010) argue, the Canadian child welfare system takes up where the residential schooling system left off, based as it is on the same "colonial discourses of Indigenous deviance and governmental trustee-ship" (p. 289). They contend that the Canadian government ignores its own role in creating the social determinants of poor health conditions for Indigenous people, while continuing to reproduce narratives about

Indigenous deficiency in terms of addictions and mental illness to justify violent interventions.

The violence inflicted by these systems on Indigenous people was described by Dylan, a Métis, queer, cisgender man in Winnipeg. He indicated that the impact of colonization and the ongoing negative effects of the ways in which child welfare agencies interact with Indigenous families were forms of structural oppression experienced by Indigenous youth:

> There's just such a long history of colonization and the impact that has on folks....I worked with primarily young people involved in the child welfare system. That system isn't able to meet their needs in terms of anything actually. The kids would have access to doctors and psychologists, but I've heard from a lot of youths whose social workers just send them to the psychologist and they don't like that, so there's a big disconnect there....It's hard for some inner-city Aboriginal street-involved young people to be sent to a doctor to help them when they've been bounced around the child welfare system, haven't seen their family in years, bounced from the streets to shelters to the streets and they're fifteen years old.

Dylan's comments resonated with those of another participant, Kyle, who shared his past experiences as an Indigenous trans youth in Winnipeg, demonstrating the violence that is inflicted by these systems. Kyle discussed being placed in a treatment centre for youth by Child and Family Services:

> Child and Family Services had put me in there because they had a shortage of group homes when I was thirteen years old. Their way of interacting with the people that didn't want to talk to a psychiatrist was by locking us in a rubber room which was the size of a bathroom. Had a camera, a hole in it, they'd leave you in there. They'd put us in these little rooms and if we don't want to talk to a counsellor about our problems, that was the ultimatum. Being put in this damn rubber room. And you know, coming from a small town and being abused by all these people and then being thrown in a psych ward and being forced to talk or we'll put you in a rubber room. "Well I don't care, I'll sit here all night if you

want, you know." I was pig-headed; everybody knew I was pig-headed. I'd sit there for hours and hours on end....After three months I got a new psychiatrist and he took me out of there. He's like, "She doesn't belong in there," and placed me in another group home finally. That was a pretty horrible experience.

Kyle's experiences show how the mental health system and child protective services play a part in ongoing violence against, and displacement of, Indigenous people. Kyle's experiences were also imbued with transphobia. After telling another psychiatrist at the same centre that he was a boy, Kyle was told he was crazy and heavily medicated. His experiences with these systems were deeply traumatizing; Kyle told me they led to "a lot of self-mutilation, like cutting and slashing my wrists and deep cutting and stuff like that." This in turn led to further medicalization, violence, and racism from mental health providers:

One doctor's pissed off 'cause one time [they] had to put seventy-two stitches to put my arm back together and he's pissed off. "I see you here every week at the [centre], I see you here every week, every second day, you know what's your problem? If you want somebody to hurt you, come here and I'll punch you in the eye."

Kyle's narrative reveals the deeply racist and transphobic character of mental health care provision and the ways in which Indigenous people are treated as worthless and disposable. This is in keeping with incidents like the 2008 death of Brian Sinclair, an Indigenous man who waited 34 hours in the emergency waiting room of a Winnipeg hospital before he died from a treatable bladder infection because he was ignored and assumed by staff to be intoxicated (Puxley, 2013). Or the 2020 death of Joyce Echaquan, an Atikamekw woman who died in the emergency room of a Quebec hospital while being subject to misogynist, racist slurs, restraints, and over-medication (Richardson & Bacon, 2021). Kyle's narrative illustrates the impact of colonization, oppression, and marginalization in the context of a racist, colonial, mental health care system. As Nelson (2012) states, "the ways in which mental health services are offered—and researched—in Canada have a foundation in one particular view of the world; that of the colonial powers who imposed this nation state on Aboriginal lands" (p. 13). And yet, these colonial foundations and contemporary implications are unacknowledged and denied in Canadian society (Nelson, 2012).

Individualizing Distress Through Pathologizing Sexualities

Participants also discussed their experiences with practitioners who pathologized their sexualities. Despite the removal of homosexuality from the DSM and resistance to the inclusion of GID (now gender dysphoria [GD]),[3] practitioners often individualized distress by positioning participants' sexualities and genders as the cause of their mental distress, rather than recognizing that living in the context of marginalization and oppression can lead to distress. In some cases this was blatant. For example, Cheyenne, a Métis, bi-queer, cisgender woman, described being assessed by a psychiatry resident in Winnipeg who "pathologized queerness and made it into this cause of disease kind of thing." During the assessment, she did not feel safe enough to disclose her sexuality. However, once he had completed the assessment she decided to come out to him. The following ensued:

> He got really upset. Not over the fact that I hadn't told him everything, but just about what it meant to be queer and what I could expect to happen in my mental health if I continued to be queer. And I was like, "Why isn't anybody…?" I literally looked at the mirror because there was a mirrored window or whatever, and I was like, "Why isn't anybody coming in here and removing this guy?" [both laugh]. "I'm sorry I didn't come out, but [laughs], you know, I don't need to hear this." And no one came. And he just kinda' wrapped it up and sputtered and was like, "K thanks, bye."

In Cheyenne's case, the pathologization of her sexuality was direct and blatant. Other participants described more nuanced scenarios in which they felt that their sexuality was being pathologized. Discussing health care practitioners and their perspectives on sexuality, Shannon, a white, queer, cisgender woman, observed, "some of them just don't have a clue. They think that it's part of your mental health problem instead of just who you are." Shannon experienced this firsthand with a psychiatrist in Winnipeg, who she said pathologized her relationships with women and seemed more eager to diagnose her after she disclosed her sexuality.

Likewise, Dana, whose psychiatrist in Winnipeg questioned her sexuality and also questioned her appearance. Dana was asked, "what are you trying to say?" in regards to her piercings and her tattoos. Her psychiatrist believed that Dana's aesthetic choices were partially at fault for her struggles, placing the blame on Dana's queer appearance rather than on the oppressive behaviours of those who discriminated against her.

Similarly, Grace, a Korean, queer, gender-fluid woman, elaborated on the ways in which her gender and sexuality had been targeted. Grace had chosen a Korean psychiatrist in hopes of creating "some sort of bridge" between herself and her parents. She found that he pathologized her appearance and behaviour for not living up to Korean cultural norms, in which children are "property," and if "an embarrassment" to their parents, a reflection of bad "parenting skills." Grace described the ways in which the psychiatrist positioned her:

> He was pointing out my physical presentation as someone who wasn't gender conformist, as someone who was queer, as someone who had piercings and tattoos. That I was an embarrassment. Which was a little hard for me to hear. And then further talked about aspects of what success meant to my family. And I said education. And I was struggling and I was trying to say that I was successful in my own way and then he said that I was not. Basically that I was a failure because I didn't have a full-time job, I wasn't married, I didn't have a home. So my entire identity to this psychiatrist was defiant.

Grace's psychiatrist used heteronormative and classist norms of appearance and success, thus deeming her a failure. As Halberstam (2011) states, "success in a heteronormative, capitalist society equates too easily to specific forms of reproductive maturity combined with wealth accumulation" (p. 2). As Grace pointed out, these norms are also racialized; she was pathologized for not living up to the expectations placed on her as a Korean woman.

As these accounts show, many practitioners pathologized non-normative sexual behaviours, identities, and experiences instead of looking at the impact of oppression. As Charlotte, a white, queer, cisgender woman, put it:

> They'd be like, "The fact that you are on the fringe and you have this queer identity is why you are feeling crazy." Instead of being like, "the context that you live in where people are homophobic douche bags is actually the supporting factor in your mental illness."

This was not the only way practitioners pathologized sexuality. Some overtly problematized participants' sexual behaviour by labelling it promiscuous.

Pathologizing Sexuality: Diagnosing Promiscuity

Diagnostic criteria for many mental illnesses include promiscuity, heightened or aggressive sexual drive, and "indiscriminate" sexual behaviour. Examples include dissociative identity disorder, borderline personality disorder, narcissistic personality disorder, antisocial personality disorder, and bipolar disorder (Diamond, 2011). These criterion are judgmental and moralistic, heavily laden with assumptions about appropriate levels of desire, numbers of sexual partners, and types of relationship within which sex should take place. Arguably, these criteria are based on heteronormative values about how much sex should be had and with whom. As Warner (1999) argues, queer culture fosters an "alternative ethical culture" that challenges sexual shame and heteronormative ways of organizing intimacy, relationships, and sexual practices (p. vii). As he claims, queer sex "is not required to be tidy, normal, uniform, or authorized by the government" (p. 35). However, some mental health care practitioners see queer forms of organizing sexual relations as a sign of mental illness.

Some participants reported being deemed promiscuous by their mental health care practitioners. Dustin, a white, queer, gay, cisgender man, described his view of the beliefs of mental health care practitioners about his having many sexual encounters with multiple partners:

> It's this idea of morality, that they are not taking care of themselves because they're not truly good people, and because of that they're having lots of sex. So it's this idea of you're a bad person, you don't care about yourself, so you're going to have lots of sex.

In this view, engaging in sex outside the bounds of a heteronormative, monogamous relationship is perceived as a sign of moral weakness and disrespect of self. Dustin explained how his sexual history was, therefore, pathologized by mental health care practitioners. However, he had his own interpretation of his behaviour:

> I've went and had lots and lots of sex with lots and lots of guys and felt pleasure and hurt that way, which is interesting. But I never physically made myself bleed because I was unhappy with who I was. So I got fucked instead. And that, to me, I've created to be normal in some interesting and weird way.

Dustin reflected a similar view to the one he attributed to practitioners in that he compared having sex with many men to self-harm. He went on to say that in the past, he did not see himself as someone who was mentally ill because he never tried to commit suicide, only thought about it. At the time of the interview, he was reconsidering this and reflecting on how having lots of sex could be seen as self harm:

> Because I have these images and understandings of mentally ill, I didn't at that time think that having lots of sex was an attribute of someone who was mentally ill. But if I was to hurt myself I would think that would be someone who was mentally ill. But I guess now thinking of it...it's understood that if someone has lots of sex, there's more chance to get HIV or to get an STI and therefore they need to take care of themselves and if they don't take care of themselves by not having lots of sex then therefore they have a problem.

In many ways, this view is aligned with the way Dustin described the perspective of mental health practitioners, linking frequent sexual activity with mental illness and an inability to care for oneself. At the same time, Dustin resisted this assessment in describing his sexual behaviour as normal, a perspective perhaps aided by critical queer norms that resist heteronormative sexual relations. Dustin resisted the pathologization of his sexual practices while at the same time naming cutting as abnormal and indicative of mental ill health, a hierarchy that he was in the midst of questioning at the time of the interview (naming it "interesting and weird").

Similarly, Chase, a white, gay, cisgender man, found that his general practitioner positioned his sexual behaviour as unhealthy and attributed it to his mental illness:

> We've talked about using it [sex] as a coping mechanism of borderline [personality disorder]. An aggressive sexual drive, seeking it out, sexual relationships that aren't necessarily healthy, be it through masturbation or through promiscuous sex. And it's been talked about like, yes, I acknowledge that I put myself in very dangerous situations. And my doctor has known this is something that you have to deal with. But we've approached it very justly, even-handedly.

Unlike Dustin, Chase did not express conflict with his practitioner, stating that he needed to be "more careful" about his sexual behaviour because the "long term negative side effects can be disastrous." Having many sexual encounters also felt unhealthy to Chase because he was often hurt by "gay men's culture" in which many men were able to "let go quickly" and not get emotionally involved. Chase went on to say that his own inability to do the same was due to having borderline personality disorder, thereby classifying both his sexual choices and his lack of being able to feel good about them as indicative of mental ill health. In this way he supported the link between mental ill health and high rates of sexual activity with multiple partners. This is not to say that the ways in which Dustin and Chase interpreted their experiences were wrong or inaccurate. Rather, I am suggesting that their perspectives were, in part, aligned with their health care practitioners' views about the links between mental illness and promiscuity.

Service providers sometimes also conflated promiscuity with non-monogamy, with the assumption being that those who had open relationships engaged in lots of sex with multiple partners. As Silver, a mixed-race, queer, cisgender person, told me,

> when I say that I'm non-monogamous and then they [mental health care practitioners] go into detective mode because I think that promiscuity is supposed to be a sign of things. I'm not promiscuous at all, but non-monogamous automatically equals [trails off]. Also it's the kind of thing where doctors assume that if you identify as such that you must be some kind of deviant. There must be something wrong with you. It's fine if you just want to meet a nice person of the same gender and settle down and adopt kids or have a puppy or something, but if you don't subscribe to that model, then automatically it's like maybe it's a sign of more mental illness [both laugh].

While Silver did not critique the concept of promiscuity, she challenged the assumption that those who were non-monogamous engaged in a lot of sexual encounters as well as the pathologization of open relationships. She drew attention to the way that homonormative relationships had attained a level of respectability in the minds of some practitioners, while other practices continued to be pathologized and linked to mental illness.

Likewise, Carter, a white, queer, trans man, described the difficulties of finding a mental health care practitioner who did not pathologize BDSM and non-monogamy. As he put it:

> I would want to be able to find somebody who I know isn't going to be like, "Well, all of your problems are related to the fact that you're non-monogamous or that you're engaged in BDSM." I have heard so many stories about that being the case.

For Carter, who identified as sex-positive, the sexually conservative values embedded in biomedical ideology were unacceptable and made it difficult for him to find an adequate service provider.

As this discussion shows, queer sexual practices and queer ways of organizing sexual relations were often pathologized by mental health care practitioners and treated as an aspect of participants' mental illness. As this discussion also indicates, some participants grappled with the internalization of sex shaming and the pathologization of queer sexual relations while others resisted such pathologization.

Pathologizing Gender Identity

The pathologizing of nonnormative gender identity was even more overt than pathologizing sexuality, partly because of the continuing inclusion of trans-related diagnoses in the DSM. For some, whether trans-identified or not, the inclusion of GID (now GD) in the DSM meant that trans-positivity and psychiatry were mutually exclusive. As Charlotte, a white, queer, cisgender woman, asked, "who is a trans positive psychiatrist? Who the fuck is that? Who's a trans positive psychiatrist? Does that exist in the world? Because we're fucking still stuck with the DSM diagnosis for that, so what the hell?" Indeed, the inclusion of diagnoses that pathologized non-normative genders had a decisive impact on trans participants, both within and apart from processes of gaining access to the technologies of medical transition.

Trans participants from Winnipeg who had navigated the mental health care system for gender identity-related needs had all done so after 2009, when Manitoba stopped referring trans people to the Centre for Addiction and Mental Health (CAMH) in Toronto.[4] Since Manitoba set up its own process for granting access to medical transition, the experience has become less pathologizing for Manitobans, as it does not take place in a psychiatric institution. The gate-keeping process was experienced as less medicalizing, and participants who had been through the process spoke positively about their experiences with the clinical psychologist who assessed their readiness for transition. Despite this, there were still concerns about having to be diagnosed with GID in order to gain access to services. As Maya said:

> I know that it's a requirement for us to get our surgery that we need the
> diagnosis. That's where it's ludicrous. I can't just say I'm trans; I have to
> get someone else to say that I'm trans. So if I make an appointment to
> see a psychologist to say, "Can you write a note to say I'm trans?" "Are
> you?" "Yes I am." "Okay." "I just told you I was."

As Maya indicated, the requirement to have one's trans identity vali-
dated by being given a diagnosis of GID (now GD) was still problematic,
although preferable to the process at CAMH.

By contrast, Torontonian participants using provincially covered
services were seen in a psychiatric institution by a psychologist and a
psychiatrist and asked invasive, irrelevant questions about their sexual
practices and desires.[5] None of the participants in this study had accessed
care through CAMH; they had paid for services privately, had not used
medical technology to transition, were not interested in transitioning, or
had accessed services in another province before moving to Toronto.

The experiences of trans people at CAMH are discussed and
critiqued within trans communities and are known to be pathologizing
and harmful in some cases. For example, Logan, a bi-racial, queer,
genderqueer person, told me that he was "afraid of them, intensely." He
went on to say:

> I've heard enough horror stories through the grapevine to be like, "I
> don't want to touch CAMH unless I was paid." And knowing my own
> ways of identifying I would fail [names a scientist at CAMH] test in a
> heartbeat. The idea of conforming to a gender role makes me incredibly
> uncomfortable and conforming to a gender performance as well.

Logan was referring to a scientist formerly employed at CAMH whose
beliefs and practices concerning trans children and adolescents have been
contested by trans activists (Tosh, 2011).[6] The test Logan referred to
is the expectation that those seeking medical transition conform to a
binary sense of gender and provide proof of having performed it over
a long enough period of time. This expectation has caused problems for
those who identify as genderqueer or challenge binary genders in terms
of gaining access to medical transition.

The horror stories Logan referred to can also affect the way that practitioners outside of CAMH are viewed. For example, Jonah, a white, bisexual, trans man, told me that he "took the whole conversation of transness off the table" with his therapist because he feared he would be pathologized for being trans. This was partially due to what he knew about CAMH's practices:

A lot of trans people, especially here in Toronto, those folks who go to CAMH, have had to deal with psychiatrists and psychologists presuming that their mental illnesses that they may have in addition to transitioning are either because of being trans or vice versa, that being trans is because of mental illness. And both of those things just cause me so much rage, for obvious reasons.

Jonah knew that the pathologizing of trans people was still rampant and wanted to avoid the possibility of hearing these views espoused by his therapist. Similarly, Trevor, another Torontonian, believed that he would always be perceived as mentally ill by any mental health care practitioner, regardless of his mental state, by virtue of being trans:

I imagine that because transsexuality has a history of pathologization that I'm already seen as having that pathology. So I'm already being viewed as mentally ill right off the get go. And it may be in my case that my anti-depressants are injectable, but that's how I feel that I'm being viewed in that moment and I don't like it.

Trevor was referring to his testosterone shots as anti-depressants, suggesting that while the technologies of medical transition may prevent him from being depressed ("my anti-depressants are injectable"), he should not be positioned as mentally ill for being trans. As this discussion shows, mental health care practitioners are often viewed with suspicion and fear by trans people because of their ongoing pathologizing of non-normative genders and are often far from being helpful resources for trans people experiencing mental distress.

As I have been arguing throughout this chapter, the biomedical model underpinning health care and social welfare practice can make for destructive power dynamics, which is compounded by lack of knowledge about, and the pathologizing of, dissident genders, sexualities, and BIPOC. As will be discussed next, biomedicalism also informs assumptions about the best way to treat mental distress and the relationship between practitioners and those seeking care.

Biomedical Methods of Managing Mental Distress: Medication as "Corrective"

The biomedical model's foundational assumption that mental illness is caused by a chemical imbalance or physiological dysfunction leads to medication as the means of "correction." Most participants who came in contact with medical professionals regarding their experiences of mental distress were met with practitioners who believed in psychiatric medication as the solution, often at the expense of addressing the social context of their distress. Sixty-two percent (23) of participants reported having taken psychiatric medication prescribed by a general practitioner or a psychiatrist, at some point. While some psychologists and counsellors also suggested medication as a means of treatment, they were unable to prescribe drugs and were more likely to also acknowledge and address the social contexts of participants' experiences.

Chemical imbalance is a widely held rationale for the prescription of psychiatric medication as a form of treatment. However, oppressive beliefs about marginalized groups can also play a role in practitioners' decisions about who requires treatment and of what sort. Fernando (2010) argues that decisions about type of treatment are rife with subtle forms of discrimination based on race. For example, anger or sadness due to the effects of "social problems" such as racism are often not appreciated by mental health care practitioners, who may, therefore, prescribe medication or ECT instead of therapy:

> If the anger is recognized as emanating from psychological or social problems, psychotherapy or "sociotherapy" (ways of influencing behaviour by manipulating the environment) may be seen as the patient's need. If the

cause of a person's depression is appreciated by the psychiatrist, psychological treatment may be used, while if it is not, ECT or antidepressant medication may be considered. (p. 112)

The many ways in which homophobia, racism, and other forms of oppression influence treatment recommendations are difficult to document. As one participant, Ameena, a South Asian, queer, cisgender woman, said:

> I had one doctor tell me that because I was South Asian I have low pain tolerance. That was really blatant racism. I think that mostly it's in the way that you get treated though. The assumptions that people make about you. Or the fact that they don't think that you need treatment or that you're exaggerating about something. And that's harder to pinpoint.

Many participants were confronted with a relentless focus on medication as a way to manage their mental distress and practitioners who were unlikely to appreciate the importance (or even the existence) of oppression in their experiences of distress. In addition, inequitable relationships between participants and practitioners made it difficult for participants to acquire the necessary support in making decisions about medication.

Psychiatrists in particular viewed medication as the only recourse. Participants who had seen psychiatrists frequently described brief encounters that ended with prescriptions for psychiatric medications, whether or not they were interested in taking them. The social contexts in which participants experienced distress were rarely considered important. For example, Dustin, a white, queer, gay, cisgender man, described his appointments with a psychiatrist as follows:

> I felt labelled. I felt constrained. I felt he [the psychiatrist] was more interested in how the medication was regulating my body and less about what I was experiencing. So "How are you sleeping?" versus, "How was you telling your parents about you coming out?" That to me is more important. I didn't really want to be on that medication in the first place. "I'm here to talk to you and that's why I'm here, but you don't want to do that." So sometimes he would end the conversations early. Sometimes

I would quickly try to say, "What do you mean by that?" And he was not happy about those kinds of conversations.

Dustin was in a consistent power struggle with his psychiatrist, and his efforts at addressing his difficulties with homophobia were rebuffed in favour of psychiatric medication as a means of treatment.

Likewise, Maya sought the help of a psychiatrist who focused solely on the prescription of medication as the answer to her feelings of depression:

> Sometimes I'd be talking to him and he'd have his eyes closed like he was sleeping. Sometimes my meetings were 10 minutes long. I would go in and it'd be, "How are you feeling?" "Not better." He'd amend the prescription and say, "We'll try this." I'd go back in the next week or two weeks. "How are you feeling?" "Still not better." "Let's try this." So it was just constantly throwing different types of drugs on me and it got to the point that I was really loopy. I stopped seeing him after a year.

Maya eventually discovered that a major cause of her depression was her inability to transition, a reason not appreciated by this psychiatrist, nor resolved through medication. Furthermore, her psychiatrist's demeanour made her feel like he was not fully present and unable to adequately support her.

Similarly, Jacy, a Métis, trans, genderqueer person, was prescribed increasing amounts and types of psychiatric medications over the course of four years. Regarding his appointments with a psychiatrist, he said,

> That person was only there to give me medication. My appointments were maybe five, ten minutes long. He would check in, "How are you doing?," summed it up quickly, and if there was something new going on he would prescribe something else for that and that was about it.

For every type of distress Jacy experienced, he was offered another type of psychiatric medication:

> It was just ridiculous. They had me on an anti-anxiety and then because I've never really been able to sleep properly they had me on sleeping pills and they also prescribed me Atavan which I was eating like fucking candy

and then I was feeling really fucking obsessive and crazy about things so they're like, "Oh, here's some Seroquel" and I had a fucking cocktail of stuff.

Jacy eventually decided to stop taking medication because it was not addressing the social context of his distress. As he said, "I feel like if there's not anything with that, if there's no support, if there's no therapy, if I'm not doing any work around it then it's just like what are they doing? It's just such a temporary solution." Like many participants, Jacy received no support in quitting his medications from the psychiatrist who was prescribing them, indicating that there is little support available for those who want to stop taking medication.

Tacit Coercion in Decision-Making About Psychiatric Medication

As Jacy's comments indicate, participants were not passive regarding treatment decisions. However, participants' agency was often compromised in decision-making regarding psychiatric medication. Coercive treatment is often understood to be explicit, such as the use of restraints and involuntary admission. But a broader understanding of coercion includes tacit coercion, also referred to as hidden, subtle, or voluntary coercion, which includes pressure to take psychiatric medication (Norvoll & Pedersen, 2016). The power dynamics implicit in the way the mental health system works influenced how much control participants felt they had over treatment decisions. Many described having contact with the mental health care system when they were in crisis and feeling desperate for help. As Morrow and Weisser (2012) argue, the Canadian mental health system is "oriented towards crisis rather than prevention, leaving those to fall through the cracks who are more stable but still need help" (p. 36). This means that when people experience a crisis, their choices are constrained, as it is more difficult to advocate for oneself or evaluate a course of treatment that is presented as the best or only option. For example, Jacy, a Métis, trans, genderqueer person, was a teenager when he first encountered the psychiatric system. He described feeling "really out of control," "really paranoid," and unable to leave his house:

> It had gone really fucking far, by the time I went in to talk to them. I was wanting to fucking kill myself and I was just completely at my wit's end. So I was just like, "Whatever you have to offer me, I'll do anything. Just make this go away." And so as soon as they offered me medication I was like, "Sure let's do it."

Many participants described a similar sense of desperation. As Jackie, a white, lesbian, cisgender woman, said, "When you're that low down and your whole world is kind of scooped from you, you're pretty much willing to go with anything that anybody could do if they tell you it will make it better." Similarly Gia, a white, gay, cisgender woman, stated,

> When you're that sick and you end up in the hospital, you kind of just go with the flow. You're not really open to debate and you're not really thinking about that kind of stuff. You just go, "Okay, take this or okay, take that." My attitude was "I'll try anything."

Additionally, the behaviour people may exhibit during a crisis is often interpreted in a sanist way; people are seen as irrational and incapable of making decisions. While it is the case that support in decision-making about treatment is often needed, this kind of behaviour can also used as justification for involuntary, forced treatment. Gia described her experiences in the hospital:

> I didn't want to get injected with a certain type of drug they wanted to try and they started threatening me and saying that they're going to get a form done or something like that. They didn't realize how sensitive I was to medications, so one of them actually made my blood pressure go down really fast.

The form Gia referred to is one that is completed to certify a person's incapacity to make treatment decisions, under Manitoba's Mental Health Act, and thus be subject to forced treatment. While this kind of involuntary treatment is often characterized as being for the patient's own good, it can have long lasting negative consequences. As Tew (2011) argues, for most people on the receiving end of involuntary treatment, it can "undermine an already fragile sense of self," create the impression that they are dangerous, alienate them from key supports, and decrease trust in mental health care professionals (pp. 152–153).

Much of the biomedical approach to psychiatric medication is predicated on the assumption not only that medication is the best way to manage distress, but that medicating those in distress is for their own good. This ideology is reflected in medical concepts like patient compliance, a term used to describe whether people take their medication as prescribed. The language of compliance, which implies submission and obedience, denies people the capability of making responsible decisions about whether or not psychiatric medication works for them. One of the more egregious examples of this kind of thinking is the development of pills containing microchips activated through interaction with stomach acid, serving the purpose of monitoring medication compliance (Halley, 2010). One such pill, Abilify MyCite, was approved for use in those diagnosed with schizophrenia and biopolar disorder in the United States in 2017 (Cornwall, 2017) but has not been approved for use in Canada. "Compliance" becomes even more disturbing when connected with evidence about who is seen as defiant, as described above. Given the existence of racism, anti-Black sanism (Abdillahi et al., 2017), and coloniality in mental health care, it is reasonable to assume that queer and trans BIPOC are more likely to be subjected to coercive measures.

The biomedical approach to psychiatric medication ignores the evidence that it can in some cases worsen mental distress. As Breggin (2008) argues, psychiatric medication can cause people to "become desperately depressed and suicidal, violently aggressive, or wildly out of control, without realizing that their medication is causing them to think, to feel, and to act in unusual and otherwise abhorrent ways" (p. 1). Indeed, the prescription of medication and the sidelining of the social context affecting the wellbeing of the participants often had adverse effects for participants.

Some participants were prescribed medication in situations that felt unsafe. As Dana, a white, Portuguese, French Canadian, lesbian, queer person, said, "you go in with a [suicide] attempt, you could go home.

So you have sutures with more meds. With more medicine to pop." She described leaving the hospital on more than one occasion after attempting suicide to go home "to myself...or to pills again or to nothing." Similarly, Charlotte, quoted above, described her first experience with the mental health system as a teenager experiencing a panic attack. She went to an urgent care centre and was seen by a psychiatrist:

> The psychiatrist talked to me for two minutes and prescribed me hundreds of tranquilizers. Like pretty much enough to kill, well, enough to kill myself for sure....What did I do after that? I took a lot of tranquilizers [both laugh]. I did [laughs]. I was a teenager. He gave me a lot of drugs. What are you supposed to do? [both laugh].

Some participants described feeling much worse on medication. Misty, a Black, queer, cisgender woman, was prescribed two anti-depressants by her general practitioner as a young adult, immediately preceding her departure for university in another city, which was far removed from her support network. She was instructed to increase her dose on her own if she felt her depression was getting worse. She said, "that's what I did. I had to see a doctor I didn't know on campus and she increased the dosage even more and I ended up in the hospital and they turned me away with a prescription for tranquilizers." Misty felt that the medication was making her feel worse but could not obtain any helpful guidance from medical practitioners. She said,

> at that point I went to a naturopath because I just had no direction in terms of medication and I had to get off of it....Obviously it [the medication] was making things worse and they just wanted to give me more.

Misty, like other participants, experienced adverse effects and did not have adequate support to make decisions about continuation, cessation, or alternatives. In many cases, the symptoms caused by psychiatric medication were unbearable for participants. Charlotte described her struggle to find a medication that worked for her:

One of them I couldn't even "get off" when I was on it. What the hell? So that was a no-go. The other one I was super rage-y. Like anger, craziness. So that was also a no-go. Like screaming crazy, screaming on [the street], like totally fucking out of control.

Similarly, Dustin, a white, queer, gay, cisgender man, described insufferable symptoms:

Taking the medication again, being on it, hating it, having sexual side effects, not being able to have sex or jerk off, being able to but not being able to enjoy it, feeling numb, feeling like a drone. I could concentrate in school, but at what cost?

For Gia, a white, gay, cisgender woman, psychiatric medication created a physical disability: "The Lithium that I was taking destroyed my thyroid. So now I have hypothyroidism forever because of that one drug. I've been toxic [liver toxicity from psychiatric medication] numerous times where I've had to go to emergency." For Gia, as for other participants, being ignored by practitioners when they expressed concern about side effects had deleterious results.

Despite the undesirable symptoms created by medication, some participants eventually decided to begin taking medication again, even when they did not want to, because practitioners portrayed medication as the only alternative. Those who refused were sometimes told they were responsible for their ill health. Dustin described feeling strong-armed into taking medication again after several years of not doing so:

Recently I actually sat in that psychiatrist's office and said, "I don't want to take pills, I've been on them, Ritalin, Paxil, I don't want to take them." After three or four conversations later, I was finally guilted. After [being] pushed and pushed and pushed to take pills, I gave in. I'm the type of person that is very much against medication. But I myself wanted to stop that conversation. And stop, I guess, the feeling of being blamed or "this can help you" or somehow believing that [laughs].

Though Dustin eventually decided to stop taking medication once again, his narrative demonstrates the impact of tacit coercion. Even participants who opposed medication and had negative experiences with it were sometimes convinced by practitioners to try again. Misty, a Black, queer, cisgender woman, eventually moved back home in order to be closer to her support network, and she then chose to resume psychiatric medication. However, she felt ambivalent about this decision:

> It's a scary thing for me because I don't really believe in it. I don't eat anything weird, I barely drink pop, so to take something like that is difficult for me. But I've gotten to a point that I'm not sure when I decide that this is something that is livable and something that is an actual illness that I need to treat. It just worries me in terms of any future relationships or work. Hopefully on a minimal dose it will help me maintain a normal life.

Misty demonstrated some confusion and hesitation, seemingly somewhat invested in the biomedical model but not entirely committed to it. Her story indicates that there is a lack of support for people who want to explore options aside from medication. Likewise, Gia, who experienced serious ramifications from psychiatric medication, felt like she had no other options:

> I became convinced that I need them and if I go off them I'm a high-risk. I don't like them, I don't want to be on them, there's medications that I'm on right now that I want to get off of. I'm at the point where I can't wait to see my doctor; I just want to stop. But you can't do that, I think....I guess they do what they do, but I don't really trust what they're doing to me. I just want to know what I'm like off them, period. I want to know if I'm the same person.

As this discussion demonstrates, many participants did not have enough support from their practitioners to make decisions that felt right to them and were instead confronted with medication as the only way to manage their distress. When medications failed to be helpful or were deleterious, many participants were left with no support or helpful direction from practitioners and no alternative ways of addressing their distress.

For a few participants, psychiatric medication had positive effects. Jackie, a white, lesbian, cisgender woman, found psychiatric medication helpful because "it really takes some of the onus of life away from you." She found that this gave her time to achieve "internal healing." She believed that in some cases psychiatric medication is "for life" because "you don't go back to work for six months and have the same thing happen again." Likewise, Levi, a white, Jewish, gay, cisgender man, found that medication was helpful for him. He told me that his brother identified as "brain damaged" from psychiatric medication and that he had "a really good reason to be afraid of medication" because pharmaceutical companies "don't give a shit" and "just need to find what they can sell." Having seen his brother's negative experiences with medication, he knew that "medications can make people sicker in the long run." Despite these views, Levi tried psychiatric medications and found that they had positive effects:

> That was my experience, getting my life back. I can work full time....And I still work full time. Never would have been able. I can't even begin to really articulate what that was like. You go out for a walk and you could smell flowers or you can feel the sun, you can feel the breeze and you're there. You're there. There's no static, you're not in a box, you're there.

As Jackie's and Levi's narratives demonstrate, it is important that people have access to medications that they find helpful. However, it is crucial that decisions are made in a non-coercive fashion. As participant narratives indicate, this would necessitate a major shift in the power imbalances between practitioners and service users and would entail shared decision-making (Morant et al., 2017).

Further, it is important to challenge the underlying assumptions about medication, or what Moncrieff et al. (2013) call the "disease-centered approach" to psychotropic medications. This approach is the most common way of understanding psychotropic medication: they work by "correcting an underlying disease of the brain" such as a chemical imbalance (Moncrieff et al., 2013, p. 214). In contrast, Moncrieff et al. (2013) propose a "drug-centered approach," that is, psychotropic drugs "produce altered mental states" that can be helpful or detrimental

(p. 215). They compare this to the useful effect that alcohol has on "very shy" people in that it lowers social inhibitions, as opposed to correcting a chemical imbalance or an "alcohol deficiency in the brain" (p. 215). They call for more analyses based on the perspectives of those who use such drugs to determine the effects they have and how they can best be used, arguing that users must be accorded much more choice in the matter (p. 230).

As Boyle (2013) notes, the drug-centred approach makes room for both "positive and negative effects of psychotropic drugs" without linking them to disease and is amenable to non-medicalized perspectives regarding mental distress (p. 9). This approach makes sense in terms of what the participants shared about positive and negative effects of drugs and supports the need for increased agency regarding the exploration of options for the management of distress. The drug-centred approach is conducive to respecting choice regarding medication use because it is the person taking medication who evaluates the efficacy of the drug rather than medical experts who believe that such drugs cure an underlying disease (Moncrieff et al., 2013, p. 229).

As discussed in Chapter 3, experiences of oppression can lead to mental distress. This chapter shows, however, that LGBTQ people experience oppression within the very system that is supposed to aid them in lessening their distress. Mental health care informed by biomedicalism makes for inequitable interactions governed by power imbalances and oppressive beliefs about sexuality, gender, and race. Racism and colonialism in mental health care made the mental health system particularly perilous for queer and trans BIPOC participants. Further, unequal relationships between practitioners and those seeking care, combined with biomedical assumptions about psychiatric medication as the most effective way to correct mental disorders left participants with inadequate choices and support about how to address their distress. This chapter demonstrates that advocating for more access to mental health treatment for LGBTQ people will not serve emancipatory aims when treatment perpetuates oppression and employs coercive strategies. The next chapter will build on this argument by examining chart documentation of 16 trans and non-binary patients on inpatient units from study two, the Cultural Representations of Gender project.

Notes

1. All names are pseudonyms.
2. According to the DSM-IV-TR, somatization disorder is diagnosed when there is no physical medical condition causing the reported symptoms or the reported discomfort exceeds the expectations of the practitioner based on evidence such as a physical examination (APA, 2000, pp. 486–490).
3. The interviews took place before GID was changed to GD in the publication of DSM-5 in 2013.
4. Prior to the launch of a trans health clinic in Winnipeg at Klinic Community Health Centre in December 2009, Manitoban trans people seeking access to transition-related surgeries were sent to the Centre for Addiction and Mental Health (CAMH) in Toronto. At the time of interviewing, the trans clinic at Klinic ran two evenings a week, with a waiting list of eight months. This clinic supports trans clients in their transition and provides prescriptions for hormones and referrals to surgeons who perform trans-related surgeries, some of which are provincially covered. At the time of interviewing, there was one clinical psychologist who provided the documentation necessary for access to hormones and surgeries. For an explanation of current options and stipulations for services covered by Manitoba Health, see https://klinic.mb.ca/health-care/transgender-health-klinic/health-care-providers/.
5. This includes questions about masturbation and pornography. At the time of interviewing, trans people seeking surgery covered by Ontario provincial insurance (OHIP) had to undergo psychological assessment and be approved for surgery at the Adult Gender Identity Clinic at CAMH. There was a waiting list of at least one year to be seen and the approval process took one to three years. CAMH has a fraught history with trans people and is heavily critiqued within trans communities, but for many years it was the only option for trans people seeking provincially covered surgeries. Those who had the means could pay for surgeries privately, though often they required at least one letter from a mental health care professional indicating readiness for surgery. For an explanation of current options and stipulations for OHIP-covered services, see https://www.rainbowhealthontario.ca/lgbt2sq-health/trans-health-knowledge-base/.
6. This scientist was employed at the now defunct Gender Identity Clinic of the Child Youth and Family Services which was closed after an external

review (Zinck & Pignatiello, 2015). This clinic for children and adolescents was distinct from the Adult Gender Identity Clinic, which is still in operation.

References

Abdillahi, I., Meerai, S., & Poole, J. (2017). When the suffering is compounded: Towards anti-Black sanism. In S. Wehbi & H. Parada (Eds.), *Reimagining anti-oppression social work practice* (pp. 109–122). Canadian Scholars Press.

American Psychiatric Association. (2000). *Diagnostic and Statistical Manual of Mental Disorders IV-TR.*

Baskin, C. (2007). Aboriginal youth talk about structural determinants as the causes of their homelessness. *First Peoples Child and Family Review, 3*(3), 31–42. https://fpcfr.com/index.php/FPCFR/article/view/48

Bennett, M., Blackstock, C., & De la Ronde, R. (2005). *A literature review and annotated bibliography on aspects of Aboriginal child welfare in Canada* (2nd ed.). First Nations Child and Family Caring Society of Canada. Retrieved August 21, 2021, from http://cwrp.ca/sites/default/files/publications/en/Abo riginalCWLitReview_2ndEd.pdf

Boxall, K., & Beresford, P. (2013). Service user research in social work and disability studies in the United Kingdom. *Disability & Society, 28*(5), 587–600. https://doi.org/10.1080/09687599.2012.717876

Boyle, M. (2013). The persistence of medicalisation: Is the presentation of alternatives part of the problem? In S. Coles, S. Keenan, & B. Diamond (Eds.), *Madness contested: Power and practice* (pp. 3–22). PCCS Books.

Breggin, P. (2008). *Medication madness: The role of psychiatric drugs in cases of violence, suicide, and crime.* St Martin's Press.

Cooper, M. B., Chacko, M., & Christner, J. (2018). Incorporating LGBT health in an undergraduate medical education curriculum through the construct of social determinants of health. *MedEdPORTAL*, 14. https://doi.org/10.15766/mep_2374-8265.10781

Cornwall, M. (2017). *The Orwellian new digital Abilify will subjugate vulnerable people across the US*. Mad in America. Retrieved August 21, 2021, from https://www.madinamerica.com/2017/11/orwellian-new-digital-abilify/

De Leeuw, S., Greenwood, M., & Cameron, E. (2010). Deviant constructions: How governments preserve colonial narratives of addictions and poor mental health to intervene into the lives of Indigenous children and families in Canada. *International Journal of Mental Health and Addiction, 8*, 282–296. https://doi.org/10.1007/s11469-009-9225-1

Diamond, S. (2011, November 17). What motivates sexual promiscuity? The psychodynamic meaning of nymphomania. *Psychology Today.* Retrieved August 21, 2021, from http://www.psychologytoday.com/blog/evil-deeds/201111/what-motivates-sexual-promiscuity

Fernando, S. (2010). *Mental health, race and culture.* Palgrave Macmillan. https://doi.org/10.1007/978-1-137-01368-2

Gaspar, M., Marshall, Z., Rodrigues, R., Adam, B. D., Brennan, D. J., Hart, T. A., & Grace, D. (2021). Mental health and structural harm: A qualitative study of sexual minority men's experiences of mental healthcare in Toronto, Canada. *Culture, Health & Sexuality, 23*(1), 98–114. https://doi.org/10.1080/13691058.2019.1692074

Giwa, S., & Greensmith, C. (2012). Race relations and racism in the LGBTQ community of Toronto: Perceptions of gay and queer social service providers of color. *Journal of Homosexuality, 59*(2), 149–185.

Halberstam, J. (2011). *The queer art of failure.* Duke University Press. https://doi.org/10.1215/9780822394358

Halley, D. (2010, December 6). *The pills have eyes: Microchipped medicine is coming.* SingularityHub. Retrieved August 21, 2021, from https://singularityhub.com/2010/12/06/the-pills-have-eyes-microchipped-medicine-is-coming/

Holthouser, A., Sawning, S., Leslie, K. F., Jones, V. F., Steinbock, S., Noonan, E. J., Martin, L., Weingartner, L. A., Potter, J., Davis, J., Eckstrand, K., & Shaw, M. A. (2017). eQuality: A process model to develop an integrated, comprehensive medical education curriculum for LGBT, gender nonconforming, and DSD health. *Medical Science Educator, 27*(2), 371–383. https://doi.org/10.1007/s40670-017-0393-5

Kanani, N. (2011). Race and madness: Locating the experiences of racialized people with psychiatric histories in Canada and the United States. *Critical Disability Discourse, 3*, 1–14. https://cdd.journals.yorku.ca/index.php/cdd/article/view/31564

McIntyre, J., Daley, A., Rutherford, K., & Ross, L. E. (2011). Systems-level barriers in accessing supportive mental health services for sexual and gender minorities: Insights from the provider's perspective. *Canadian Journal of*

Community Mental Health (revue Canadienne De Santé Mentale Communautaire), 30(2), 173–186. https://doi.org/10.7870/cjcmh-2011-0023

Menzies, R., & Palys, T. (2006). Turbulent spirits: Aboriginal patients in the British Columbia psychiatric system, 1879–1950. In J. Moran & D. Wright (Eds.), *Mental health and Canadian society: Historical perspectives* (pp. 149–175). McGill-Queen's University Press.

Moncrieff, J., Cohen, D., & Mason, J. (2013). The patient's dilemma: An analysis of users' experiences of taking neuroleptic drugs. In S. Coles, S. Keenan, & B. Diamond (Eds.), *Madness contested: Power and practice* (pp. 3–22). PCCS Books.

Morant, N., Azam, K., Johnson, S., & Moncrieff, J. (2017). The least worst option: User experiences of antipsychotic medication and lack of involvement in medication decisions in a UK community sample. *Journal of Mental Health, 27*(4), 322–328. https://doi.org/10.1080/09638237.2017.1370637

Morrow, M., & Weisser, J. (2012). Towards a social justice framework of mental health recovery. *Studies in Social Justice, 6*(1), 27–43.

Nelson, S. (2012). *Challenging hidden assumptions: Colonial norms as determinants of Aboriginal mental health.* National Collaborating Centre for Aboriginal Health. Retrieved August 21, 2021, from https://www.ccnsa-nccah.ca/docs/determinants/FS-ColonialNorms-Nelson-EN.pdf

Norvoll, R., & Pedersen, R. (2016). Exploring the views of people with mental health problems on the concept of coercion: Towards a broader socio-ethical perspective. *Social Science & Medicine, 156*, 204–211. https://doi.org/10.1016/j.socscimed.2016.03.033

Nowaskie, D. (2020). A national survey of US psychiatry residents' LGBT cultural competency: The importance of LGBT patient exposure and formal education. *Journal of Gay & Lesbian Mental Health, 24*(4), 375–391. https://doi.org/10.1080/19359705.2020.1774848

Obedin-Maliver, J., Goldsmith, E. S., Stewart, L., White, W., Tran, E., Brenman, S., Wells, M., Fetterman, D. M., Garcia, G., & Lunn, M. R. (2011). Lesbian, gay, bisexual, and transgender-related content in undergraduate medical education. *Journal of the American Medical Association, 306*(9), 971–977. https://doi.org/10.1001/jama.2011.1255

Pilling, M., Howison, M., Frederick, T., Ross, L., Bellamy, C. D., Davidson, L., McKenzie, K., & Kidd, S. A. (2017). Fragmented inclusion: Community participation and lesbian, gay, bisexual, trans, and queer people with diagnoses of schizophrenia and bipolar disorder. *American Journal of Orthopsychiatry, 87*(5), 606.

Puxley, C. (2013, August 29). Brian Sinclair: Man who died after 34-hour Winnipeg hospital wait was assumed to be "sleeping it off" after vomiting. *Toronto Star*. Retrieved August 21, 2021, from http://www.thestar.com/news/canada/2013/08/29/brian_sinclair_man_who_died_after_34hour_winnipeg_hospital_wait_was_assumed_to_be_sleeping_it_off_after_vomiting.html

Richardson, L., & Bacon, S. (2021, May 14). Joyce Echaquan's family describes seeing her "tied up like an animal" in Joliette hospital bed. *APTN News*. Retrieved August 21, 2021, from https://www.aptnnews.ca/national-news/joyce-echaquans-family-describes-seeing-her-tied-up-like-an-animal-in-joliette-hospital-bed/

Rutherford, K., McIntyre, J., Daley, A., & Ross, L. (2012). Development of expertise in mental health service provision for lesbian, gay, bisexual and transgender communities. *Medical Education, 46*, 903–913. https://doi.org/10.1111/j.1365-2923.2012.04272.x

Tew, J. (2011). *Social approaches to mental distress*. Palgrave Macmillan. https://doi.org/10.1007/978-1-349-92463-9_8

Tosh, J. (2011). "Zuck off!" A commentary on the protest against Ken Zucker and his "treatment" of childhood gender identity disorder. *Psychology of Women Section Review, 13*(1), 10–16.

Vermette, L. (1988). The 33 years of the lost Indian walk. In B. Burstow & D. Weitz (Eds.), *Shrink resistant: The struggle against psychiatry in Canada* (pp. 117–120). New Star Books.

Yellow Bird, P. (2004). Wild Indians: Native perspectives on the Hiawatha Asylum for Insane Indians. Retrieved August 21, 2021, from http://www.patdeegan.com/pdfs/PeminasManuscript.pdf

Warner, M. (1999). *The trouble with normal: Sex, politics, and the ethics of queer life*. Harvard University Press.

Zinck, S., & Pignatiello, A. (2015). *External review of the gender identity clinic of the child, youth and family services in the underserved populations program at the centre for addiction and mental health*. TransAdvocate.com. Retrieved August 20, 2021, from https://www.transadvocate.com/wp-content/uploads/GIC-Review-26Nov2015-TA1.pdf

5

The Biomedical Model in Practice II: Psychiatric Inpatient Chart Documentation on Trans and Non-Binary People

This chapter builds on the argument established in Chapter 4 regarding the subjective and discriminatory character of biomedical practice by examining chart documentation from study two regarding 16 trans and non-binary patients on inpatient units in a psychiatric hospital in Ontario. My analysis of the charts shows that the logic of cisnormativity underpinned practitioners' documentation practices, resulting in persistent problems in the way trans and non-binary people were treated in psychiatric settings. Cisnormativity governed institutional means of collecting data regarding patient demographics, such as the inconsistent use of correct pronouns, names, and gender identities, which in turn facilitated basic problems in recognizing the humanity of trans and non-binary people. Further, I argue that practitioners employed a cisnormative, transmisogynist lens in their descriptions of patients' appearance and mannerisms, resulting in the pathologizing of trans and non-binary gender expression, especially trans femininities. Practitioners also displayed a significant lack of knowledge about trans and non-binary life, which resulted in the individualizing of structural inequities and the pathologizing of trans and non-binary experiences of marginalization and violence. This chapter further demonstrates that advocating for more

© The Author(s), under exclusive license to Springer Nature Switzerland AG 2022
M. D. Pilling, *Queer and Trans Madness*,
https://doi.org/10.1007/978-3-030-90413-5_5

access to mental health treatment will not serve emancipatory aims when treatment continues to reinforce cisnormative, damaging assumptions about trans and non-binary life, identities, and ways of being.

Demographics

As described in more detail in the Introduction, this chapter draws on data from a study in which 161 psychiatric inpatient charts were analysed for content related to gender, sexuality, race, class, and disability. In this chapter, I focus on the 16 charts of trans and non-binary people. I could not rely on the institution's demographic data to provide an accurate representation of patients' sexuality and gender because of the institution's cisnormative practices for gathering such data, as will be discussed in more detail below. In order to create a coherent description of the gender demographics, I employed a trans-positive lens to affirm trans and non-binary ways of being and resist the institution's imposition of cisnormative and transphobic understandings of gender. I performed a close reading of each chart, looking for clues as to how patients self-identified in terms of gender. This was an exceedingly difficult task, given the muddled, cisnormative, and transphobic ways in which trans and non-binary patients were described by most practitioners and the problematic institutional practices for gathering such data. This difficulty in identifying the sexuality and gender of trans patients is noteworthy because patients' self-identification should be clearly evident in the charts.

In creating my description, my goal was to categorize trans and non-binary patients' gender identity in a way that was both trans positive and more accurate than the many labels imposed by the psychiatric institution. However, in the absence of data on self-identification, my demographics are bound to contain inaccuracies and should not be seen as definitive. Each chart contained conflicting information about patients' gender identities with only two exceptions. Two people were consistently perceived by all practitioners as cisgender, heterosexual men, but the following description categorizes them as transfeminine people because of various indications in their chart that this was likely the case.[1] The 16 charts discussed in this chapter comprise those of two Black, trans women, one Indigenous, trans woman, eight white, trans women/transfeminine people,[2] one white, trans man, and four white, non-binary people. In the case of four people, sexuality was erroneously recorded as transgender. For the others, one was recorded as bisexual, one as asexual, two as queer, five as "do not know," two as heterosexual,[3] and one chart was left blank. The patients ranged in age from 21 to 61, with a mean age of 33. Three people were employed, nine were on social assistance, one had no income, two preferred not to answer, and one person's financial information was not recorded. Four of the 16 people had an income between $15,000 and $29,000, and the rest made below $15,000, or their income was not recorded. This places all of the people for whom financial information was recorded well below the poverty line in the city in which they resided.

The demographics described above raise two questions: why is the sample predominantly trans women, transfeminine, and non-binary people, and why is the sample made up of mostly white people? The latter is perhaps easier to answer. The larger sample of 161 from which these 16 charts are drawn were sampled from four units within the psychiatric institution. However, the charts of trans and non-binary people were mostly (15/16) sampled from the general psychiatric unit. The demographics from the larger sample indicate that the majority of patients (70%) on the general psychiatric unit were white.[4] This may explain why the smaller sample of 16 was also predominantly (81%) white people.

The predominance of transfeminine and non-binary people in the sample speaks to their heightened visibility within the institution in contrast to transmasculine people. As Serano (2013) argues, transfeminine people are highly scrutinized and "culturally marked" because of a combination of misogyny and transphobia (transmisogyny), whereas transmasculine people are often invisiblized (p. 50). Psychiatry pathologizes femininity generally and gender-nonconforming femininity in particular (Tosh, 2016), resulting in the heightened scrutiny and pathologizing of transfeminine and non-binary people in the psychiatric institution. It is possible that some transmasculine people may choose to avoid detection as trans within the institution as a survival strategy and that this may be harder to do as a transfeminine person because of their hypervisibility due to transmisogyny.

Institutionalized Cisnormativity in Health Care

Cisnormativity is the privileging of cisgender identities, bodies, and ways of being as natural, normal, and authentic (Bauer et al., 2009; Hudson, 2019). It is a system of power that treats cisgenderism as the default and enables erasure of, and violence against, trans and non-binary people (Boe et al., 2020). Cisnormativity upholds a binary understanding of sex (male and female) and gender (men and women) and expects and enforces enduring congruence between sex assigned at birth, gender identity, and cultural expectations of masculinity and femininity (Borba & Milani, 2017). For example, those assigned male at birth are assumed to become men who are aligned with cultural expectations of masculinity in appearance and behaviour and who will remain so throughout their lives. At the heart of cisnormativity lies an ahistorical Eurocentrism that denies that the binary sex/gender system is a colonial construct violently imposed on Indigenous peoples, thereby attempting to erase precolonial and current Indigenous gendered ways of being (Picq & Tikuna, 2019).

As I am using it here, cisnormativity also refers to the cis-centric view of the world that allows cisgender people to be unaware of, or to underestimate the frequency, severity, and extent of transphobia all around them. Cisnormativity allows cisgender people to be surprised when confronted with an example of transphobia or to engage in wilful denial, disbelief, or minimizing because they do not personally experience transphobia. Transphobic incidents are thereby portrayed as being much less prevalent than they are, as a one-time mistake, or due to some other factor (a misunderstanding, a bad day, etc.) rather than seeing transphobic incidents for what they are: examples of harm perpetuated within a pattern of systemic violence endemic in society.

Cisnormativity is so ubiquitous that it is a common sense way of thinking or, as Bauer et al. (2009) state, "cisnormative assumptions are so prevalent that they are difficult at first to even recognize" (p. 355). In health care systems, cisnormativity is embedded within "texts and forms, protocols and policies, and institutional infrastructure" that are "set up in ways that assume cissexuality and are thus often inappropriate for trans identities, trans bodies, and trans lives" (p. 355). Institutionalized cisnormativity in health care has serious implications for the health of trans and non-binary people. It results in the ongoing erasure of the needs and existence of trans and non-binary people and allows for the "continued assumptions that systems do not need to be adapted to be trans-appropriate and that trans people can be dealt with on an individual basis" (p. 356). This creates inaccessible and ineffectual health care for trans and non-binary people. It also enables and normalizes the dehumanization of trans people in encounters with health care systems and providers. Cisnormativity is heightened within a psychiatric context where anything non-normative in the strictest sense is reconfigured as abnormal, resulting in heightened scrutiny and pathologizing. As Tosh (2017) suggests, the ever-growing list of disorders in the DSM indicates that within psychiatry "the concept of normality has become so constrained that it represents an idealized form of white, middle class, heterosexual, cisgender masculinity that is impossible to attain" (p. 263).

While all trans and non-binary people are affected by cisnormativity, some may feel its effects more sharply. Cisnormativity elevates trans and non-binary people who are more readily perceived as cisgender over those who are not (Boe et al., 2020). Trans and non-binary people who are perceived as being most closely aligned with cisgender norms of appearance and behaviour are "more readily legible" and are often seen as more legitimate than those who are less likely to be perceived as cisgender (Boe et al., 2020, p. 158). It should not be assumed that being perceived as cisgender ("passing") is desirable for every trans and non-binary person; there are many for whom it is not or for whom it is incidental (not a goal). There are also many trans people for whom some, or all, of the technologies of medical transition are out of reach for financial or other reasons. This is especially true for those on the transfeminine spectrum, for whom there are often greater costs. Given that the majority of the 16 people included in the sample were transfeminine and non-binary people living in poverty, it can be assumed that both medical technologies of transition (e.g., hormones, surgery) and non-medical means of gender expression or transition (e.g., make-up, clothing) were difficult to access for those who desired them. This means that they may have been even more likely to be seen as straying from cisgender norms and, therefore, as abnormal and abject in the context of the cisnormative psychiatric institution. As this indicates, cisnormativity impacts trans and non-binary people in different ways along lines of gender and class. Cisnormativity also intersects with other systems of oppression including racism. The confluence of cisnormativity, racism, misogyny, and transphobia results in specific experiences of discrimination and violence against trans women of colour who are impacted by racist transmisogyny (Hudson, 2019) and Black trans women who experience transmisogynoir (Bailey & Trudy, 2018). The following will illuminate the ways in which cisnormativity was evident in the charts of trans and non-binary patients, highlighting intersections with other forms of oppression where possible.

Cisnormative Institutional Practices for Capturing Patient Demographics

The presence of cisnormative practices in charting are evident from examining the form used by the institution to collect patient demographic data. The following will outline some of the elemental problems with this form. This is not the sole focus of this chapter, and my analysis is, therefore, not exhaustive.[5]

The institution employs a multidisciplinary initial assessment (MDA) form to collect a robust amount of patient demographic data including age, gender, language preference, immigration and citizenship status, race, religion, housing type, disability, sexual orientation, income amount and type, and professional and informal supports—but not pronouns. Following triage, the MDA is completed by a number of different practitioners including nurses, social workers, physicians, and residents. Many of the demographic questions, including those regarding gender and sexual orientation, are completed using a drop-down menu with pre-set options. The first two questions on the MDA are age and gender. However, these two questions were consistently left blank in most charts, including those of cisgender patients in the larger dataset.[6] One possible reason for the omission of information regarding gender identity could be because some practitioners were unaware that there was a difference between gender and sexual orientation. This was evidenced by the fact that some practitioners responded to the question about sexual orientation by choosing the option labelled "Other (please specify)" and typing in a gender identity, such as "transgender from female to male." Another reason for the omission may be because the charts also contain a highlighted bar that appears at the top of the screen with select information about the patient, including (but not limited to) name, allergies/sensitivities, age, gender, medical record number, and attending physician. The information in the highlighted bar concerning patients' age, name, and gender are populated from the patient's Ontario health card (rather than the MDA), which is entered by non-medical staff when people arrive at the institution. It is possible that practitioners assume that the age and gender fields on the MDA are redundant, given this information already appears at the top of the screen.[7]

This practice of completing patient name and gender using data from government-issued identification is problematic for many trans and non-binary people, who for legitimate reasons may not have identification that lists their correct name and gender. This cisnormative practice assumes that a patient's name and gender on identification aligns with the patient's current name and gender, and supports and facilitates the misgendering of trans and non-binary patients. Highlighting the legal name and gender at the top of the chart increases the likelihood that practitioners will misgender patients whose name or gender have changed but whose identification has not. It may also create problems for trans and non-binary people whose identification has changed to reflect their correct name or gender since the last time they visited the institution (for a further discussion of similar issues, see Deutsch et al. [2013]). While the MDA provides a place to include correct gender, as aforementioned this question on the MDA was rarely completed, including in all of the 16 charts in the sample discussed in this chapter.

Further, the drop-down menu that is meant to capture patient gender includes limited options. The question reads: "What is your sex/gender?

Check <u>ONE</u> only: female, male, intersex, trans–female to male, trans–male to female, prefer not to answer, do not know, other (please specify)."[8] The forced selection of only one option belies identifying as more than one of the available options (for example, some people are both intersex and trans). While some trans people use the terms "female to male" and "male to female," there is a growing preference for "trans man" and "trans woman." The MDA does not include any gender options for those who identify beyond the binary,[9] including non-binary, genderfluid, genderqueer, and agender.[10]

Notably, the MDA also does not include an option to provide correct pronouns[11] or a name that differs from one recorded on the health card.[12] These omissions and the other problems I have described are based on cisnormative logic that precludes the existence of trans people and contributes to their institutional erasure (Bauer et al., 2009; Namaste, 2000) as well as creating conditions for the violence of misgendering to flourish. However, these problems do not begin and end with the institutional means of gathering demographics. The charts offer many opportunities for practitioners to write free-form narratives, unrestrained by drop-down menus with preset options. The charts, therefore, contain myriad gendered references throughout, written by all manner of professionals including doctors, nurses, social workers, pharmacists, recreational therapists, and nutritionists. The rest of this chapter will explore this in more detail.

The Basics: Correct and Respectful Language

As discussed, the institutional means of collecting gender demographics are such that trans and non-binary patients are misgendered and erased in the process of gathering such data. An analysis of the charts of transgender and non-binary patients further reveals that most practitioners hold deeply cisnormative understandings of gender and lack even the most basic awareness of correct and respectful language in referring to and addressing trans and non-binary people.

For example, the charts contain many uses of the word transgendered (instead of trans or transgender), and is often employed as a noun, which is dehumanizing. The chart of Alyssa,[13] a white trans woman, includes the following description: "29 year old single male to female transgendered, lives in an apartment alone" (instead of trans woman, for example).[14] Further, with the exception of the two charts of trans-feminine people who were consistently assumed to be cisgender men, every chart contained various and usually conflicting language to describe patients' gender identity. This suggests that many, if not most, practitioners made assumptions about the ways in which patients identified, rather than asking patients for the correct terms. It also suggests that practitioners do not always read the rest of the chart (see also Gibson, 2021).

This phenomenon was especially pronounced in the charts of non-binary people. For example, Morgan, a white non-binary person, was consistently misgendered throughout their chart. They were referred to by a nurse as "a transgender from male to female," by a doctor as a "man with gender identity issues, prefers to be called 'Morgan'" and by a pharmacy student as "Morgan ([birth name]) [age] year old unspecified gender admitted voluntarily." Likewise, Spencer, a white non-binary person, was incorrectly referred to as a "single female who goes by the name 'Spencer'" by a nurse in the intake note. The next day, a social worker noted:

> Spencer indicated a difficulty in sleeping and experiencing stressful life circumstances. Spencer identifies as gender binary and asks to be addressed as "they." Pt [patient] explains the gender identity is something "They" were aware since an early age but only recently discovered while attending some AA meetings. Pt indicates "they" have a supportive network of friends in the trans community.

The social worker was unfamiliar with the correct term, non-binary (or gender non-binary), instead referring to Spencer as "gender binary." The meaning of the social worker's second sentence is unclear, likely indicating a lack of knowledge regarding gender identity. The social worker seemed unaware that they/them pronouns are commonly used by non-binary people and puts them in scare quotes, casting doubt on the authenticity of gender-neutral pronouns. The social worker went on to place they/them pronouns in scare quotes five more times throughout this note, eight times in the next case management note, and five times in the third case management note.[15] Later the same day a doctor wrote: "[birth name], who identifies as Spencer because she [sic] is non-gender binary, presented to [name of hospital] ED [emergency department] yesterday describing distress and anxiety." Like the social worker, the doctor did not know the term non-binary (or gender non-binary), instead referring to Spencer as "non-gender binary," and misgendering Spencer by using their birth name and the pronoun she. In this same note, the doctor referred to the name Spencer as the middle name on their health card and used the pronoun she throughout, demonstrating great confusion and lack of care. Spencer's chart contains many similar examples of misgendering, such as the pharmacy student who noted that "'Spencer' is a [age] year old woman."

Incorrect and Inconsistent Use of Pronouns

As many of the examples discussed above also indicate, most of the charts are riddled with inconsistent and incorrect pronoun use by practitioners of all kinds. This may be a common problem in medical institutions, as suggested by a study that shows inconsistent use of pronoun and/or name in 43.2% of charts of transgender youth receiving psychiatric inpatient care in the United States (Bieber et al., 2020). Haven, a white, non-binary person who was most often referred to as a "trans male" or a "transgender male" but who was also correctly referred to sometimes as non-binary, was frequently misgendered with incorrect pronouns. One doctor wrote: "Haven is a [age] year old gender non-binary person. She [sic] has a long history of addiction to alcohol and a variety of other substances. They prefer to be referred to with the gender neutral pronoun 'they.'" The doctor correctly noted that Haven was non-binary but used the pronoun she to begin the note, despite explicitly noting that Haven's pronouns were they/them. Another doctor wrote that Haven was a "transgender male who is referred to as 'they.'" Like the social worker who documented in Spencer's chart, this doctor placed they/them pronouns in quotation marks, indicating unfamiliarity with gender-neutral pronouns and questioning their authenticity. This also occurred in Morgan's chart, a white, non-binary person: a social worker noted that Morgan "would like to use pronoun 'they.'"

Many of the charts contained inconsistent pronoun use even within the same sentence, often making it difficult to discern the writer's meaning. For example, a doctor wrote the following in Jade's (a white, trans woman) chart: "Worries re his [sic] mom…. She cannot reach her for almost a year, still hoping she would contact him [sic]." Later in the same note, the doctor wrote: "She is asking to spend this weekend, at least, on a secure environment, in which he [sic] feels she will not execute any SA [suicide attempt]." Likewise, a nurse noted that Nia, a Black, trans woman, was a "transgendered male to female" and then wrote: "Patient comes into the ER today complaining of anxiety and 'losing his [sic] mind.' Patient reports she was admitted…on Tuesday for the same complaint." The lack of care shown in using incorrect pronouns is especially grievous given the ease of editing the written word; one can only imagine how frequently patients must be verbally misgendered.

Some practitioners demonstrated a blatant disregard for patients' identity and pronouns. Armen, a white, trans man, was consistently misgendered throughout his chart. On intake, a doctor identified Armen as a "[age] year old transgendered female to male" and then wrote the following: "She reports that she is sexually active with her fiancé and her LMP [last menstrual period] was 4 days ago. She states that she likes to be in relationship with a male and 'hates' to be called a female." Despite noting Armen's feelings about being misgendered ("'hates' to be called a female"), the doctor chose to use female pronouns throughout the note. That this constituted harm and created distress seemed lost on this doctor who simultaneously documented that they were engaging in "alliance building" with the patient.

Deadnaming: Denying Trans Subjectivity and Self-Determination

Calling a trans person by the (usually gendered) name assigned to them at birth once they have chosen another name that better aligns with their gender is sometimes referred to as deadnaming. Turton (2021) argues that deadnaming is a "potentially injurious speech act" and "akin to the utterance of a slur" (p. 44). Deadnaming should be understood as

> a discursive practice through which trans identities are invalidated in an effort to maintain the normative belief that the only natural human subject is one that exhibits a binaristic, predictable and permanent alignment between a corporeal sex assigned at birth (male or female), a gender identity (boy/man or girl/woman) and a gender expression (masculinity or femininity). (p. 43)

Practitioners employed cisnormative practices that placed primacy on patients' dead names and questioned the authenticity of their real names.[16] Patients' real names were often placed in scare quotes, referred to as aliases, and/or included in the chart after the use of dead names, for example: "[dead name] 'Nia' [last name] is a [age] year old male to female transgendered person." Institutional practices such as writing patient names on their doors and on a large whiteboard in a common area facilitated the public deadnaming of trans and non-binary patients. Amber, a white, trans woman, experienced public deadnaming on the unit, which was humiliating and distressing. This was described by a nurse as follows:

> Pt [patient] is requesting to be called and to write her name on the board only Amber not [dead name]. Pt stated that it was written in the daytime and pt was upset. Emotional support provided. Will pass the message to the next shift. Continue to monitor and provide support. Maintains on close observation.

Despite the nurse's stated intention to inform the nurses on the next shift, it was evident that staff continued to publicly deadname Amber.

Two days later a nurse recorded the following: "Compliant with her medications. Well groomed. Pleasant and polite on approach. Pt reports feeling frustrated when her name is on the assignment board as '[dead name]' rather than 'Amber.' Responding well to encouragement and support."

Similarly, Haven, a white, non-binary person, was publicly dead-named on the unit. A doctor wrote the following: "Haven told me, they feel unsafe on the medical ward because their name was written as '[dead name]' on the door and they would like it changed to Haven." Later that same day, a nurse noted:

> [Patient] reported that "I am upset the staff are calling me [dead name] I want to be called Haven," reassurance and support provided and patient felt supported, came for lunch and went back to bed with no contact to co-patients remains isolative in "their" room. Patient reassured and supported and encouraged to engage in unit activities, currently have a visit from "their" sister.

The nurse indicated a lack of familiarity with they/them pronouns by using scare quotes, which also called into question the authenticity of Haven's pronouns. The nurse noted that Haven was not socializing ("no contact to co-patients") and referred to them as "isolative," without making any connections to the fact that Haven had been publicly dead-named and consistently misgendered, making the unit an unsafe place for socializing.

Deadnaming is a form of violence, and its negative impact should not be underestimated. World Professional Association for Transgender Health (WPATH) indicates that using the wrong name for trans patients harms the therapeutic alliance between patients and practitioners and puts patients at risk of verbal and physical violence from other patients (Deutsch et al., 2013). The distress caused by deadnaming is especially important to consider in the context of the psychiatric institution, where patients are already experiencing heightened states of distress, suicidality, and loss of autonomy. Turton (2021) writes that deadnaming undermines trans people's self-determination and argues that

deadnaming is aptly termed, not only because it reanimates a past identity that is "dead" to the subject upon whom it is imposed, but because
the aim of deliberate deadnaming is to bring about the "death" of the
subject's self-identity—to suspend its social reality, to reassert the borders
of cisnormativity and to deny the subject the status of legitimate speaker
on their own behalf. (p. 59)

Within the psychiatric institution, cisnormativity is compounded by
sanism, which works to deny patients' agency and positions practitioners
as experts on patient's lives. In other words, psychiatric patients are
already positioned as unreliable and illegitimate narrators, even regarding
their own lived experience, while practitioners are positioned as experts
who know best. Deadnaming by practitioners in a psychiatric context
compounds sanism to further deny trans and non-binary subjectivity
and autonomy. As an American study of trans and gender nonconforming youth found, those "who were able to use their chosen names in
multiple contexts reported fewer depressive symptoms and less suicidal
ideation and behavior" (Russell et al., 2018, p. 505). In a psychiatric
institution where people are already feeling distressed and suicidal, the
violence of deadnaming and misgendering is especially toxic and must
be understood as a form of harm and dehumanization.

Pathologizing (Trans)Gender: Cisnormative and Transmisogynist Patient Descriptions

Thus far I have discussed what I refer to as "the basics" because addressing
the problems I have described would be a starting point that could (and
should) be addressed with consistent training and changes to institutional practices and policies. Consistent use of correct names, pronouns,
and gender identity is a basic level of respect and acknowledgement of
humanity that should be afforded every person who enters any institution (whether psychiatric or otherwise). There is no acceptable excuse
for cisnormative institutional practices that harm and dehumanize trans
and non-binary people through consistent misgendering. However, these
necessary institutional changes would only address practices that are

overt; there are also deeply embedded, insidious problems that are more difficult to address.

One such problem is the way in which practitioners pathologize trans and non-binary identity, gender expression, and ways of being. The change of gender identity disorder (GID) to gender dysphoria (GD) in the DSM-5 was supposed to signal the end of pathologizing trans-genderism due to the shift in focus in the diagnostic criterion from pathologizing identity to pathologizing distress. However, as Tosh (2017) argues, gender dysphoria is just the "latest name change" in a long line of diagnoses that have pathologized gender nonconformity (p. 62). Of note, there were two charts in which gender identity disorder was still used, even though these charts were written after the publication of the DSM-5 (2013) and one additional chart that listed "Gender Identity Transitional Issues" under diagnosis. Further, gender-related diagnoses are just one way of pathologizing trans people. As discussed repeatedly throughout this book, pathologizing distress is not necessarily better than pathologizing identity. Further, a change in diagnostic name or criterion in the DSM is different from a change in practitioner perspective and practice. Cisnormativity in health care services means that "transgender people more readily experience cultural messages of what constitutes an appropriate gendered body than cisgender people" (Boe et al., 2020, p. 160). An analysis of the charts revealed that practitioners pathologized gender nonconformance, especially trans femininities, and made assessments of trans and non-binary patients' gender expression using a cisnormative, transmisogynist lens.

Sloane's chart displayed the most overt example of pathologizing gender nonconformance because it was linked directly and exclusively to psychosis; practitioners did not even consider that Sloane may have been trans or non-binary. Sloane, a white, transfeminine person, was consistently perceived as a cisgender man by all practitioners. On admission, a doctor wrote:

> Mr. [last name] has schizoaffective disorder with prominent psychosis and prominent mood sxs [symptoms]. In the past he has been admitted in highly agitated states where he would frequently explode in anger and when he was so disorganized that he was incoherent. At his most psychotic he also used to wear women's clothes and make-up.

Sloane's sartorial and aesthetic choices ("women's clothes and make-up") were seen as an indication of psychosis rather than an authentic exploration or expression of gender identity. This reflects longstanding ideas about psychosis and gender nonconformance that conflate the two, especially in the case of trans femininities. In Sloane's discharge note, a doctor stated the following:

> On discharge Mr. [last name] presented as a muscular male who looked his stated age who was dressed in [type of clothing] attire, which was primarily male in gender. The patient still identifies himself as female but agrees that he has a male persona and male genitalia. He was approachable and cooperative.

The doctor presented Sloane's female identification as illogical and incongruent with Sloane's appearance (muscles, 'male' clothing), presentation ("male persona"), and body ("male genitalia"). In so doing, the doctor employed what could be called the holy grail of cisnormativity: the erroneous assumption that genitals determine gender (and sex), an assumption that has been dismantled by trans and intersex communities and 30 years of Gender Studies scholarship (Bornstein, 1995; Butler, 1990/1999; Fausto-Sterling, 2000; Kessler, 1998; Vaid-Menon, 2020). The doctor's use of the phrase "male persona" reveals another hallmark of cisnormativity: the imperative that everyone must present a consistent, coherent, and recognizable binary gender. In other words, Sloane's identification as female was seen as an impossibility given their "persona" and gendered presentation. In fact, some trans and non-binary people choose to present in variously gendered ways from day to day, and some may feel like they have to present as one gender in certain situations for safety reasons (such as at work or in a psychiatric hospital). However, gender expression can be uncoupled from gender identity; one's outward appearance does not always determine or indicate gender identification (Vaid-Menon, 2020).

Further, the doctor employed the transmisogynist belief that in order to identify and be perceived as a woman one must do so "well," that is, in compliance with cisnormative standards of what a woman should look like. This notion was further reinforced by the doctor's description of Sloane's appearance in the same discharge note:

Initially, during his hospital stay, he was quite irritable and difficult to approach, as well as extremely disorganized and bizarre-looking. He was not groomed, had very unkempt dreadlock hair, and was often wearing a combination of male and female clothing, with copious amounts of rouge applied inappropriately on his face.

The doctor's comments indicate the assumption that in order to be seen as female one must adhere to cisnormative standards of femininity. The doctor portrayed Sloane as doing femininity badly ("bizarre-looking") by wearing both 'men's' and 'women's' clothes and an incorrect amount ("copious amounts") of rouge, applied in the "wrong" way ("applied inappropriately").

There is also the question as to why the doctor found it necessary and relevant to document Sloane's gendered appearance at all. It is clear that the doctor linked Sloane's gendered presentation to mental wellness (and illness). In other words, the doctor found such details pertinent in the context of describing how Sloane was doing in terms of mental health. In comparing Sloane's appearance on intake versus on discharge, the doctor seemed to suggest that there was an increase ('improvement') in Sloane's gender conformity, which was equated with an improvement in Sloane's mental health symptoms. In contrast to the description of Sloane on intake, the doctor noted that on discharge Sloane "was bearded and dressed in men's clothing and was not wearing make-up. He was polite, cooperative and not agitated hostile or yelling." The doctor linked a perceived increase in gender coherence and alignment with sex assigned at birth with an improvement in Sloane's comportment and mental wellness, positioning gender nonconformance as pathological. It is important to note that there was no documented effort to ascertain whether Sloane wanted to explore gender identity and no gender identity resources were offered, such as connections to local trans-affirming community organizations. There was also no indication that trans or non-binary gender identity was considered by the practitioners at all. This is deeply troubling, given Sloane's history of multiple suicide attempts. Sloane was discharged feeling "stressed and down" and experiencing "passive suicidal wishes" and auditory hallucinations telling Sloane to die by suicide.

As shown in Sloane's chart, the confluence of misogyny and transphobia (transmisogyny) means that transfeminine people are seen as bizarre or pathological for displaying characteristics culturally associated with femininity. This phenomenon was also evident in the charts of other transfeminine and non-binary people. Practitioners frequently passed judgment on patients' gendered appearance and clothing, especially in the context of feminine gender expression. For example, in the chart of Orion, a white, non-binary person, a doctor wrote: "Clean dressed and reasonably groomed, though style slightly bizarre." Later that same day, a doctor noted: "Unique style. Pants seem like they may be made for women. Appropriate for weather." Like Sloane's style choices, Orion's were seen as "bizarre" and "unique," based on cisnormative and transmisogynist logic that dictates that that clothing has a (binary) gender and that those assigned male at birth should wear clothing culturally associated with masculinity.

Similarly, Irie, a Black, trans woman, was described by a doctor as "strangely dressed and poorly groomed." A nurse described Irie's appearance as follows: "Pt. [patient] is wearing a long blonde wig and a short skirt dressed like a woman but unshaven. Mood is labile." The nurse's note employs a cisnormative lens that indicates an incongruence between Irie's facial hair and her clothes, suggesting that Irie failed at expressing femininity in an acceptable (read: cisnormative) way. On more than one occasion, a practitioner commented on the pitch of Irie's voice, stating that she spoke in "falsetto," as one nurse noted: "Loud and speaking in falsetto while interacting with staff." The use of the word falsetto is telling. Falsetto is defined as "an unnaturally or artificially high-pitched voice or register, especially in a man" (www.dictionary.com/browse/falsetto). The nurse's use of "falsetto" reveals a transmisogynist logic that positions Irie as a man 'posing' as a woman, using an 'artificial' register. This logic was further evidenced in notations written by a nurse on two occasions that Irie "moves in an exaggerated feminine manner" and that "he [sic] was wearing a skirt, a wig, and moved in a feminine manner."

Irie's chart also displayed the confluence of misogyny, transphobia, and anti-Black racism (transmisogynoir) (Bailey & Trudy, 2018). Irie was variously described as "loud," "labile," and sometimes "threatening," reflecting oppressive beliefs about Black people as disruptive and threatening. Further, a higher level of coercion and control was displayed in Irie's chart. Irie was admitted involuntary and determined to be incapable of making treatment decisions. Her chart also made reference to administering sedating drugs "with security present," a phrase that signals tacit coercion (see Zaheer, 2021). On intake, a doctor noted that practitioners should "use PRNs liberally,"[17] a directive that seems to have been followed as Irie was often so drugged as to be incoherent and slurring her words: "Client was very sedated…and could not engage in meaningful conversation. He [sic] was up briefly for dinner, but ate poorly due to his [sic] sedative state. He [sic] went back to his room and he [sic] has been sleeping till the present time." Similarly, another nurse recorded the following: "Pt. [patient] found with multiple hand-written notes strewn about his [sic] bed. Notes are non-sensical. He [sic] is unable to answer other questions due to sedation." The same note stated that Irie's speech was "slurred, slowed." As a Black, trans woman, Irie's gender transgressions contributed to practitioners' transmisogynoirist perception of her as out of control, pathological, and in need of containment (for further discussion of Irie's chart, see Daley [2021] and Pilling [2021]).

Pathologizing Trans and Non-Binary Life: Individualizing Structural Inequities

In addition to pathologizing patients' gender expression, practitioners displayed a lack of familiarity with common concerns, barriers, and experiences of trans and non-binary people. For example, practitioners expressed doubt that Haven, a white, non-binary person, was able to self-inject hormones and questioned their knowledge of their dosage. Those with a basic familiarity with trans and non-binary life know that many trans and non-binary people who take hormones do so by self-injecting, often on a weekly or bi-weekly schedule. Depending on how long someone has been taking hormones, they may have been self-injecting for years. If someone has been self-injecting on a weekly schedule for even just one year, that person would have self-administered a hormone shot 52 times. And yet, a nurse marvelled at Haven's ability to self-inject, while simultaneously misgendering them: "self administered her [sic] testosterone injection with a considerable skill."

This lack of familiarity with trans and non-binary life sometimes meant that structural inequities were individualized and seen as indicative of patient deficits. For example, those with a basic understanding of trans and non-binary life know that public washrooms can be a major site of anxiety for trans people because of the frequent transphobia and gender policing that happens in these spaces. The gendering of public space according to a binary framework and the discrimination trans people face within gendered spaces is the result of structural inequity, in which the transphobic fears of cisgender people are prioritized over trans people's right to exist in public space. This issue often comes to the attention of mainstream media via discussions of transphobic "bathroom bills" in the United States (Lopez, 2017), though Canada has not escaped this transphobic discourse (Lum, 2020).

Practitioners seemed unaware of how using washrooms in the psychiatric institution could impact trans and non-binary patients. Nia, a Black, trans woman, was described as having "deficits" in her ability to self care because "He [sic] also reports he was scared to shower at the hospital as he felt someone would come into the shower." Likewise, Jade, a white, trans woman, expressed concern about using the women's washroom, which were recorded by a doctor as follows: "She has troubles with assertiveness. She spoke about not being allowed to use the female bathroom which she is welcome to use. The gender neutral bathroom is out of services due to enteric surveillance." Jade's reluctance to use the women's washroom was characterized as her fault ("troubles with assertiveness") rather than a common and reasonable concern due to transphobia. In this way, the doctor also sidestepped any responsibility on the part of the institution to provide an accessible substitute for the gender-neutral washroom that was out of service.

In another example, Alyssa, a white, trans woman, expressed concern about her employment prospects, including fear that sex work was the only way she could generate income. A doctor noted that Alyssa was "terrified" of her current workplace going out of business because "she feels that she will be lost if she cannot work at [place of work]. She sees that her only alternative would be to prostitute as 'no one will hire her for being transgendered.'" Alyssa's concern did not seem to be taken seriously or treated as reasonable, despite the fact that it was documented elsewhere in Alyssa's chart that she had worked as an "escort" in the past and despite the widespread discrimination trans women face in the workforce (Bauer et al., 2011; Irving, 2015).

Pathologizing Survival: Reconfiguring Experiences and Effects of Marginalization as Delusions and Paranoia

Cisnormativity also allowed practitioners to be ignorant of the widespread nature of street harassment and transphobia, and to reconfigure these experiences as delusions and paranoia. As scholars have argued, mental health practitioners generally do not investigate whether there is any empirical basis for the beliefs they deem delusional or paranoid (Georgaca, 2004; Harper, 2004). Rather, practitioners make these decisions based on common sense and "taken for granted social and cultural assumptions" (Harper, 2004, p. 56). As I argue elsewhere, such common sense beliefs include oppressive ideologies such as rape culture and anti-Black racism, resulting in patient experiences of, and responses to, sexual violence being reconfigured as delusional thinking (Pilling, 2021). Likewise, cisnormativity is a form of common sense that underpins practitioners' understandings of trans and non-binary patients' experiences of transphobia and other forms of oppression. As Harper (2011) argues, "when we use the notion of paranoia to diagnose others we may obscure the real causes of their distress, locating it instead in faulty brain mechanisms, rather than out there in a frequently hostile world" (p. 64).

This phenomenon was particularly visible in the charts of Black and Indigenous trans women, showing the intersections of cisnormativity with the logics of settler colonialism, anti-Black racism, and transmisogyny. For example, Cindi, an Indigenous trans woman experienced transphobic harassment prior to her hospitalization. On the first day of her admission, a doctor noted the following:

> Pt [patient] is originally from [name of province] but moved to [name of Canadian city] to "get away from homophobia." She recently moved to supportive housing...in hopes that the residents at her old building would stop harassing her....She still hears them mocking her from the apartments beside her saying "[transphobic and homophobic slurs]." She reports that she is certain she is being followed because her window has a few bullet holes in it and her deadbolt lock was broken a few days ago. She does not feel there could be another explanation for her experience.

The doctor believed that the other explanation for Cindi's experience was that she was paranoid and having delusions of persecution. The doctor did not seem to entertain the notion that Cindi could be experiencing harassment, despite the fact that trans women of colour experience high rates of violence and Indigenous women in Canada are targeted and murdered at rates at least 4.5 higher than for other women (Saramo, 2016). The narrative throughout Cindi's chart constructed her experiences of harassment and transphobic discrimination as delusions of persecution and paranoia, showing that the service providers were far removed from the lived realities of an Indigenous, trans woman living in poverty. There was no awareness that colonization created the conditions in which Cindi lived, or of poverty, transphobia, and homophobia as traumatic and informing her experiences of distress. Rather, her thoughts were deemed delusional and paranoid and were seen as indicative of psychosis. On the second day of her admission, a doctor noted that these delusions indicated that Cindi may be presenting with "possible psychosis" and started her on anti-psychotic drugs. The day before Cindi was discharged, a doctor noted: "Patient remains psychotic, and believes gangs harassing her at her home, but not in hospital. Wanting transfer to inpatient rehab. Plans on discharge to shelter tomorrow." Despite noting that Cindi's concerns were specifically related to the harassment she experienced in her neighbourhood ("but not in hospital"), Cindi's account was seen as delusional and symptomatic of psychosis. No effort was made to help Cindi with her housing safety, and she was discharged to a shelter because she did not feel safe returning home. Based on Cindi's request for a transfer to inpatient rehabilitation, a referral was made to a rehabilitation facility. Her distress regarding harassment and suicidality was treated with anti-psychotic medication, suggesting that the problem was seen as being with Cindi's brain, rather than with a transphobic society. Before discharge, Cindi was placed on a depot (injected) anti-psychotic, making it more difficult for her to discontinue this medication if she so desired. Of note, Cindi was frequently misgendered with incorrect pronouns and referred to as a man by various practitioners, which was a source of further (unacknowledged) distress and revictimization by the psychiatric institution (for further discussion of Cindi's chart, see Daley [2021] and Gibson [2021]).

Similarly, Nia, a Black, trans woman, was seen as having paranoid delusions based on her accounts of street harassment. On the first day of her admission, a doctor wrote:

> [She] feels like there are people out there, "black people" who drive around and follow him [sic], rip up her wigs, her clothes. She feels that perhaps they are committing hate crimes against her, for "dressing up" and to confirm her "health condition" by finding pills. She also believes that these problems happen only after she dresses up, and posts pictures on Facebook. She sees 3 cars, one was white, and she took the licence plate down.

The doctor was sceptical that Nia was harassed "only after she dresses up," indicating a lack of awareness that Nia would be at much greater risk of violence when presenting in a visibly feminine way and that Black trans women experience disproportionate levels of violence, including murder (Preston, 2020). Ironically, the doctor dismissed Nia's experiences of harassment while simultaneously inflicting harm by misgendering her. The doctor further indicated that Nia was "Increasingly fearful, that she is being persecuted for her transgender orientation and HIV positive status, despite an undetectable viral load," as if discrimination stops when viral load is undetectable. Nia was characterized as being paranoid and suffering from paranoid delusions. This was repeated by a doctor the following day: "paranoia being followed because of being trans and HIV," which became a refrain throughout the chart. The doctor deemed that Nia was experiencing first-episode psychosis with paranoid delusions and started her on anti-psychotic medication.

Documentation by a nurse the following day provides some insight into Nia's perspective about why she sought assistance from the institution, which differed greatly from the practitioners' narratives: "Client reported 'I am here because need help with my anxiety, people have been breaking into my house, now it is the sixth time and nobody believes me, they think am crazy.'" Nia repeatedly requested a letter from the physician to support her request for a transfer to alternate housing. Upon discharge, a letter was provided as follows:

> To whom it may concern: [birth name] [last name] [[DOB]) was admitted to our psychiatric inpatient unit from [date range]. She attributes an important reason for the admission being her distress about her neighbours harassing her and would like to request transfer of housing. Sincerely, [name and credentials].

Notably, the doctor did not make any statement of support regarding Nia's concerns about harassment ("she attributes") or explicitly support her request for a transfer of housing. It is questionable as to how much support this letter provided in Nia's quest for different housing to escape harassment. No further efforts to help Nia with her housing situation were made. There is no documentation regarding the use of her birth name on the letter and whether this was requested by Nia. This is an important consideration given that the use of a name (whether birth name or current name) can inadvertently disclose trans identity, depending on the circumstances.

Like Cindi, Nia experienced repeated home invasions and street harassment. The two women also struggled with unemployment, suicidality, substance use, a diagnosis of HIV, and poverty. These are essentially the compounded "symptoms" of structural inequities and interlocking systems of power and domination such as settler colonialism, anti-Black racism, white supremacy, and transmisogyny. But within the normative psychiatric institution, these issues were characterized as individual deficits signalling psychosis, and the solution was anti-psychotic medication. Both women named what they needed (help with housing and substance use), and these requests were either denied or addressed half-heartedly in a manner that suggested that they were seen as secondary to medication.

Of note, practitioners showed readiness to pathologize all manner of experiences and behaviours, not just those of street harassment and transphobic discrimination. For example, Patricia, a white, trans woman with a long history of homelessness, was documented as having previously suffered a broken hip for which she had not received any medical treatment. Patricia used a cane to walk, and her gait was frequently noted to be "abnormal" and "unsteady" because of her untreated injury. Despite this, a nurse noted that "Pt [patient] engages in a shuffling side-step to ambulate, which may be as a result of OCD/delusional symptoms." Patricia's way of walking was seen as potentially indicative of OCD and delusional thinking, as opposed to the way she was able to move given her disability. Patricia was also documented by a doctor as being paranoid because she refused assistance in looking for subsidized housing: "She does not want to apply even for waiting lists, as she does not want this team or anyone else having any information about her, likely related to paranoia." Patricia was being held involuntarily in the institution, having previously been declared incapable of consenting to treatment and injected with medications against her will. She contested this at Ontario's Consent and Capacity Board and lost the hearing. Given the lack of respect for her agency and bodily autonomy, it makes sense that she would not want to share any personal information with the team that could facilitate her location being known. And yet this was characterized as "likely related to paranoia."

This is not to say that the experience of paranoia and delusions do not exist. But in some cases, like those described above, practitioners may be denying a current or recent reality. In other cases, they may be denying past experiences by attributing patients' paranoia and delusions to a disordered brain rather than exploring how it may reflect past experiences of violence. In both cases, the existence and impact of violence against trans people were erased. This is also illustrated in the chart of Kirsten, a white, trans woman. Kirsten was described by a doctor as "clearly having command hallucinations to kill herself and paranoid delusions" regarding men harassing her in the street. In her discharge note, a doctor wrote:

> She explained that sometimes she has spells, when under stress, in which she does not want to talk to anybody, becomes suicidal, hears voices of men for a few minutes and "visualizes in her mind" men in black. She recognizes that these are men that have attacked her in the past and when under stress she can imagine them.

According to the doctor, Kirsten suggested that she was not experiencing harassment at the moment but because of past experiences of being harassed, she could hear the voices of the men who had attacked her. As I argued in Chapter 3, it is vital to insist on the intelligibility of mental distress, behaviours, and thoughts that seem abnormal through focusing on "the idea that people's feelings and actions are consonant with their past and present experiences" (Boyle, 2011, p. 41) rather than attributing distress to physiological dysfunction. As Johnstone (2011) argues, the experience and impact of traumatic experiences can become "concealed and lost…behind a mountain of individualizing and pathologizing psychiatric theories" (p. 108). As she further claims, it is not helpful to ask "can trauma cause psychosis?" More helpful questions include, "what are the ways in which people (can) react to trauma? Do these (routinely) include some of the experiences we refer to as 'hallucinations' and 'delusions'?" (pp. 108–109). Posing such questions requires a paradigm shift that forces acknowledgement of the existence of violence and, as discussed, has very different implications for addressing the distress that results from violence.

Why Does It Matter?

The problems I have described in this chapter all point to trans and non-binary people being more likely to be seen as bizarre and pathological in appearance, behaviour, and beliefs because of the ways that cisnormativity shapes practitioner understandings of gender and trans and non-binary lives. Why does this matter? There is, of course, the obvious: that trans and non-binary people should be treated with respect rather than as bizarre anomalies. Health care practitioners have a duty to respectfully treat all patients regardless of their familiarity with trans and non-binary identities and the existence and impact of structural barriers and inequities. Lack of familiarity should not be seen as an excuse for treating people poorly; it should be seen as an indication of the necessity to acquire appropriate education. Further, my analysis of the charts indicates that psychiatric institutions are unsafe places for trans and non-binary people and disrupts the idea that changing or removing gender identity-related diagnoses from the DSM will stop the pathologization of trans and non-binary people. As Kirby (2014) states,

> instead of being trans people who creatively survive transphobia, we are trans people with anxiety disorders, anger disorders, bipolar [disorder], schizophrenia. Our basic identities are less and less considered a "mental illness," but our strategies for surviving are being taken out of context and individualized as "mental illnesses." (p. 163)

It is also important to consider whether the pathologizing of trans and non-binary people increases the risk of coercive 'treatment.' Of note, seven of the 16 patients arrived at the institution involuntarily through a Form 1, which is an application by a physician for psychiatric assessment. Under the Mental Health Act of Ontario, this form can be completed by any physician who has examined a patient within the previous seven days.[18] Patients must meet the criterion outlined on the form, which, broadly speaking, includes actual or potential harm to self or others or a lack of competence to care for self. A Form 1 results in involuntary institutionalization for up to 72 hours for psychiatric assessment, which cannot be contested. Of the seven people admitted on a Form 1, five were subsequently converted to voluntary status while two were not and continued to be held against their will. Coercive treatment is problematic because of the violation of bodily autonomy. Further, involuntary hospitalization has been shown to increase the risk of attempting suicide following institutionalization (Jordan & McNiel, 2020). It is also important to note that even 'voluntary' admissions can be tacitly coerced (Norvoll & Pedersen, 2016) when patients are told that they will be held involuntarily if they do not consent to a 'voluntary' admission. Voluntary patients are often also afforded more 'privileges' (such as being allowed to go outside for accompanied or unaccompanied walks), which can be an incentive to agree to a 'voluntary' admission.

Relatedly, the problems I described in this chapter matter because the impact of the violence I have described does not dissipate when trans and non-binary people exit the institution. Trans and non-binary people carry the impact of their experiences at the institution with them. Trans and non-binary people who end up at the institution are in states of heightened distress and instead of receiving help they are subjected to harm. Twelve of the 16 people (75%) reported some kind of current or historical relationship to suicide, including those who were either suicidal at the time of admission, became suicidal during their admission, or had considered or attempted suicide in the past. Of the four who did not report any relationship to suicide, two people refused to answer any questions about suicidality and suicide attempts, and two people reported no history of suicide attempts or suicidal ideation but had engaged in self-harm prior to their admission. This is consistent with a study of trans Ontarians, which found an extremely high rate of suicidal ideation and attempts with 35.1% considering suicide and 11.2% having attempted it in the previous year (Bauer et al., 2015). This study also found that "lower self-reported transphobia…was associated with a 66% reduction in ideation…and an additional 76% reduction in attempts among those with ideation" (Bauer et al., 2015). Trans and non-binary people who present at the institution wanting to die should not be met with dehumanizing and pathologizing treatment that will surely contribute to their distress. In the words of Deegan (2008), "help isn't help if it's not helpful. Help that is not helpful can actually do harm."

Cisnormativity normalizes transphobic oppression both within and outside the psychiatric institution and allows cisgender people to underestimate both the prevalence and the impact of these institutionalized problems. My analysis of the charts reveals a combination of interrelated problems that are both overt and insidious. Overt problems with cisnormative institutional data collection practices enable and support the dehumanization of trans and non-binary people through constant misgendering. Making changes to these overt problems will require a multi-pronged approach. It is obvious that intake procedures and forms need to change to reflect the existence of trans and non-binary people. However, all staff (non-medical and medical) also require ongoing training to be able to understand how to respectfully elicit the correct information and record it in an accurate way. It is evident that all staff also require training on how to consistently respect self-identification in chart documentation as well as verbally when speaking face-to-face with patients and when discussing patients with coworkers. This will require a shift in many practitioners' cisnormative worldviews that govern ideas about how women, men, and non-binary people should appear and behave.[19]

While these changes are necessary, there is a danger that only the most basic and overt problems will be addressed, allowing the institution to claim leadership in diversity, equity, and inclusion while simultaneously continuing to pathologize trans and non-binary people in insidious ways. The problems I have described, such as pathologizing trans and non-binary gender expression and the lived experience of structural inequities, are deeply embedded in and interrelated with the issues of the biomedical model described in Chapter 3, such as the lack of respect for agency and bodily autonomy. My analysis of the charts illustrates the danger of advocating for better access to psychiatric treatment when the institution continues to reinforce cisnormative, damaging assumptions about trans and non-binary life, identities, and ways of being as well as fails to respect bodily autonomy. Psychiatric institutions need to be made less unsafe for trans and non-binary people who want to, or are forced to, access them, but there is also an urgent need for different options than the ones that are currently available. The next chapter will explore change within and outside mental health care systems, including community strategies such as collective care and mutual aid, and how this provides pathways forward, away from the psy complex.

Notes

1. For example, a referral to a gender identity clinic.
2. Given the lack of information about self-identification, I use the more expansive term transfeminine in cases where it was unclear if the person would have identified as a trans woman. I use transfeminine as an umbrella term to capture all those who identified on a feminine gender spectrum in contrast to their sex/gender assigned at birth but who may or may not have

identified as a trans woman. In doing so, I also recognize that the terms transfeminine and transmasculine can be seen as replicating a binary view of gender.

3. As noted, two patients were recorded as being cisgender, heterosexual men, whereas I have categorized them as transfeminine people. This misdesignation may mean that they were not heterosexual (for example, if they were attracted to women, they may have identified as queer or lesbian).

4. This in turn raises the question of why the patients in the general psychiatric unit were mostly white. In contrast, our sample from the unit that treated people with a diagnosis of schizophrenia and other related diagnoses, had a disproportionate number (47%) of Black patients. This resonates with the work of scholars who explore the racialization of diagnoses and argue that Black people are disproportionately diagnosed with schizophrenia (Fernando, 2010; Metzl, 2009). For a more detailed discussion, see Daley and Pilling (2021).

5. Readers looking for further information on common problems with cisnormativity in electronic medical records and how to ameliorate them should consult the recommendations created by the World Professional Organization for Transgender Health electronic medical record working group (Deutsch et al., 2013).

6. A physician who worked at the institution at the time of writing in May 2021 claimed that this was no longer the case.

7. Informal communication in May 2021 with a physician who works at the institution confirmed that this could be a factor. The reasons are multifactorial and perhaps best assessed by observing what happens in practice. However, in my experience of delivering curriculum regarding trauma-informed care and 2SLGBTQ competence to multi-disciplinary service providers in health care and social services, many service providers are uncomfortable asking clients about gender identity and sexual orientation and feel ill equipped to do so respectfully despite their best intentions.

8. At time of writing in May 2021, the MDA had undergone minor changes. The question now reads: "What is your gender?" and no longer asks the practitioner to check only one option (but only one option can be selected). The gender option of two-spirit has been added.

9. This is not to suggest that trans man and trans woman are binary identities for everyone who self-identifies in this way, though they are for some. Further, some trans men and women also identify as non-binary.

10. This should not be seen as an exhaustive list.
11. I deliberately use the word "correct" instead of the commonly employed word "preferred," which undermines authenticity. The word preferred is rarely used to describe pronouns used by cisgender people. Pronouns used by trans and non-binary people are not a preference—they just are.
12. At time of writing in May 2021, the highlighted bar at the top of the chart included a new field for "name used" following the name on the health card. There is no similar update to the MDA.
13. All names are pseudonyms, and the pseudonyms replace the patients' actual names in quotations from their charts.
14. The terms female to male and male to female have fallen out of popularity in the last 10 years but are sometimes still employed especially by trans people over the age of 40, which is why it is important to ask people about self-identification and then consistently use the correct term.
15. Because of the way the charts were anonymized, it is unknown if it was the same social worker who completed all three documentation examples. The painstaking use of scare quotes throughout is remarkable given the haste with which most notes seem to be written; spelling mistakes and acronyms abound.
16. I deliberately use the designation "real" instead of "preferred" to subvert cisnormative logic that positions legal names as authentic and chosen names as a preference that can be disrespected or ignored. It can be financially prohibitive and difficult to obtain identification with the correct name and gender marker (Beattie, 2021), and the state should not be the arbiter of trans personhood.
17. PRN, or pro re nata, refers to medication given when necessary. It was often employed in the charts to refer to benzodiazepines (tranquilizers).
18. More research is needed to determine whether trans people are disproportionately detained involuntarily, though it may be challenging to assess given the issues with demographic data collection, as described in this chapter.
19. At the time of writing in May 2021, I met with one person in a leadership position at the institution who indicated a commitment to making changes to the intake form.

References

Bailey, M., & Trudy. (2018). On misogynoir: Citation, erasure, and plagiarism. *Feminist Media Studies, 18*(4), 762–768. https://doi.org/10.1080/146 80777.2018.1447395

Bauer, G. R., Hammond, R., Travers, R., Kaay, M., Hohenadel, K. M., & Boyce, M. (2009). "I don't think this is theoretical; this is our lives": How erasure impacts health care for transgender people. *Journal of the Association of Nurses in AIDS Care, 20*(5), 348–361. https://doi.org/10.1016/j.jana.2009.07.004

Bauer, G. R., Nussbaum, N., Travers, R., Munro, L., Pyne, J., & Redman, N. (2011). We've got work to do: Workplace discrimination and employment challenges for trans people in Ontario. https://transpulseproject.ca/wp-con tent/uploads/2011/05/E3English.pdf

Bauer, G. R., Scheim, A. I., Pyne, J., Travers, R., & Hammond, R. (2015). Intervenable factors associated with suicide risk in transgender persons: A respondent driven sampling study in Ontario, Canada. *BMC Public Health, 15*, 525. https://doi.org/10.1186/s12889-015-1867-2

Beattie, S. (2021). Transgender woman says getting gender-affirming ID in Ontario is an "impossible struggle." *CBC News.* Retrieved August 22, 2021, from https://www.cbc.ca/news/canada/toronto/ontario-transgender-identific ation-gender-1.6117750

Bieber, E. D., Voort, J. L. V., Croarkin, P. E., Vonn Drehle, C. T., Simon, S. M., Hopp, B. N., Heil, H. M., & Romanowicz, M. (2020). Documentation practices for transgender youth admitted to an inpatient psychiatric unit. *Journal of Psychiatric Practice, 26*(2), 153–159. https://doi.org/10.1097/PRA.0000000000000453

Boe, J. L., Ellis, E. M., Sharstrom, K. A., & Gale, J. E. (2020). Disrupting cisnormativity, transnormativity, and transmisogyny in healthcare: Advancing trans inclusive practices for medical family therapists. *Journal of Feminist Family Therapy, 32*(3–4), 157–175. https://doi.org/10.1080/08952833.2020.1848051

Borba, R., & Milani, T. M. (2017). The banality of evil: Crystallised structures of cisnormativity and tactics of resistance in a Brazilian gender clinic. *Journal of Language and Discrimination, 1*(1), 7–33. https://doi.org/10.1558/jld.33354

Bornstein, K. (1995). *Gender outlaw: On men, women, and the rest of us.* Routledge.

Boyle, M. (2011). Making the world go away, and how psychology and psychiatry benefit. In M. Rapley, J. Moncrieff, & J. Dillon (Eds.), *De-medicalizing misery: Psychiatry, psychology and the human condition* (pp. 27–44). Palgrave Macmillan.

Butler, J. (1990/1999). *Gender trouble: Feminism and the subversion of identity.* Routledge.

Daley, A. (2021). Narrating genders in psychiatric inpatient chart documentation. In A. Daley & M. D. Pilling (Eds.), *Interrogating psychiatric narratives of madness: Documented lives* (pp. 57–86). Palgrave Macmillan.

Daley, A., & Pilling, M. D. (2021). Introduction: Psychiatric documentation, power and violence. In A. Daley & M. D. Pilling (Eds.), *Interrogating psychiatric narratives of madness: Documented lives* (pp. 1–31). Palgrave Macmillan.

Deegan, P. (2008). When help is not helpful. *Addiction and Recovery News.* Retrieved August 22, 2021, from https://addictionandrecoverynews.wordpress.com/2008/05/12/more-from-pat-deegan-2/

Deutsch, M. B., Green, J., Keatley, J., Mayer, G., Hastings, J., Hall, A. M., Blumer, O., Brown, S., Cody, M. K., Fennie, K., Hall, A. M., Mayer, G. S., Moscoe, G., St. Claire, R., River Stone, M., Wilson, A., & Wolf-Gould, C. (2013). Electronic medical records and the transgender patient: Recommendations from the World Professional Association for Transgender Health EMR Working Group. *Journal of the American Medical Informatics Association, 20*(4), 700–703. https://doi.org/10.1136/amiajnl-2012-001472

Fausto-Sterling, A. (2000). *Sexing the body: Gender politics and the construction of sexuality.* Basic Books.

Fernando, S. (2010). *Mental health, race and culture.* Palgrave Macmillan.

Georgaca, E. (2004). Factualization and plausibility in delusional discourse. *Philosophy, Psychiatry, & Psychology, 11*(1), 13–23. https://doi.org/10.1353/ppp.2004.0037

Gibson, M. F. (2021). Forming the chart: Texts, actions, and differences. In A. Daley & M. D. Pilling (Eds.), *Interrogating psychiatric narratives of madness: Documented lives* (pp. 33–56). Palgrave Macmillan.

Harper, D. J. (2004). Delusions and discourse: Moving beyond the constraints of the modernist paradigm. *Philosophy, Psychiatry, & Psychology, 11*(1), 55–64. https://doi.org/10.1353/ppp.2004.0041

Harper, D. J. (2011). The social context of paranoia. In M. Rapley, J. Moncrieff, & J. Dillon. (Eds.), *De-medicalizing misery: Psychiatry, psychology and the human condition* (pp. 53–65). Palgrave Macmillan.

Hudson, K. D. (2019). (Un)doing transmisogynist stigma in health care settings: Experiences of ten transgender women of color. *Journal of Progressive Human Services, 30*(1), 69–87. https://doi.org/10.1080/10428232.2017.1412768

Irving, D. (2015). Performance anxieties: Trans women's un(der)-employment experiences in post-Fordist society. *Australian Feminist Studies, 30*(83), 50–64. https://doi.org/10.1080/08164649.2014.998455

Johnstone, L. (2011). Can traumatic events traumatize people? Trauma, madness and "psychosis." In M. Rapley, J. Moncrieff, & J. Dillon (Eds.), *De-medicalizing misery: Psychiatry, psychology and the human condition* (pp. 99–109). Palgrave Macmillan.

Jordan, J. T., & McNiel, D. E. (2020). Perceived coercion during admission into psychiatric hospitalization increases risk of suicide attempts after discharge. *Suicide and Life-Threatening Behavior, 50*(1), 180–188. https://doi.org/10.1111/sltb.12560

Kessler, S. J. (1998). *Lessons from the intersexed*. Rutgers University Press.

Kirby, A. (2014). Trans jeopardy/Trans resistance: Shaindl Diamond interviews Ambrose Kirby. In B. Burstow, B. LeFrançois, & S. Diamond (Eds.), *Psychiatry disrupted: Theorizing resistance and crafting the (r)evolution* (pp. 163–176). McGill-Queen's University Press.

Lopez, G. (2017). Anti-transgender bathroom hysteria, explained. *Vox*. Retrieved August 22, 2021, from https://www.vox.com/2016/5/5/11592908/transgender-bathroom-laws-rights

Lum, Z. (2020). Peter MacKay campaign walks back calling trans rights legislation a "bathroom" bill. *HuffPost News*. Retrieved August 22, 2021, from https://www.huffingtonpost.ca/entry/peter-mackay-email-transgender-rights_ca_5eac81eac5b6b0b1b53596d4

Metzl, J. (2009). *The protest psychosis: How schizophrenia became a Black disease*. Beacon Press.

Namaste, V. (2000). *Invisible lives: The erasure of transsexual and transgendered people*. University of Chicago Press.

Norvoll, R., & Pedersen, R. (2016). Exploring the views of people with mental health problems' on the concept of coercion: Towards a broader socio-ethical perspective. *Social Science & Medicine, 156*, 204–211.

Picq, M. L., & Tikuna, J. O. S. I. (2019). Indigenous sexualities: Resisting conquest and translation. In C. Cottet & M. L. Picq (Eds.), *Sexuality and translation in world politics* (pp. 57–71). E-International Relations

Publishing. Retrieved August 22, 2021, from https://www.e-ir.info/2019/08/20/indigenous-sexualities-resisting-conquest-and-translation/

Pilling, M. D. (2021). Sexual violence and psychosis: Intersections of rape culture, sanism, and anti-Black sanism in psychiatric inpatient chart documentation. In A. Daley & M. D. Pilling (Eds.), *Interrogating psychiatric narratives of madness: Documented lives* (pp. 137–163). Palgrave Macmillan.

Preston, A. M. (2020). The anatomy of transmisogynoir. *Harper's Bazaar*. Retrieved August 22, 2021, from https://www.harpersbazaar.com/culture/features/a33614214/ashlee-marie-preston-transmisogynoir-essay/

Russell, S. T., Pollitt, A. M., Li, G., & Grossman, A. H. (2018). Chosen name use is linked to reduced depressive symptoms, suicidal ideation, and suicidal behavior among transgender youth. *Journal of Adolescent Health, 63*(4), 503–505.

Saramo, S. (2016). Unsettling spaces: Grassroots responses to Canada's missing and murdered Indigenous women during the Harper government years. *Comparative American Studies: An International Journal, 14*(3–4), 204–220. https://doi.org/10.1016/j.jadohealth.2018.02.003

Serano, J. (2013). *EXCLUDED: Making feminism and queer movements more inclusive.* Seal Press.

Tosh, J. (2016). *Psychology and gender dysphoria: Feminist and transgender perspectives.* Routledge.

Tosh, J. (2017). Gender non-conformity or psychiatric non-compliance? How organized non-compliance can offer a future without psychiatry. In M. Morrow & L. Halinka Malcoe (Eds.), *Critical inquiries for social justice in mental health* (pp. 255–282). University of Toronto Press.

Turton, S. (2021). Deadnaming as disformative utterance: The redefinition of trans womanhood on Urban Dictionary. *Gender & Language, 15*(1), 42–64. https://doi.org/10.1558/genl.18816

Vaid-Menon, A. (2020). *Beyond the gender binary.* Penguin Workshop, Pocket Change Collective.

Zaheer, J. (2021). Documenting restraint: Minimizing trauma. In A. Daley & M. D. Pilling (Eds.), *Interrogating psychiatric narratives of madness: Documented lives* (pp. 111–135). Palgrave Macmillan.

6

Creating Social Change: The Emancipatory Promise of Queer and Trans Madness

This chapter explores change both within and outside of the mental health care system. Based on the analysis of participant narratives from study one and chart documentation from study two presented in Chapters 4 and 5, respectively, I discuss changes within the mental health care system that would make it more liveable for 2SLGBTQ people. Drawing on participant narratives about collective care and mutual aid, I also explore the ways mad queer and trans people can and do engage in ways of responding to mental distress outside of the mental health system. This includes a discussion of barriers to such approaches, including the need to address intra-community oppression. I then outline some responses to acute distress and crisis created by and for queer and trans people that reject coercive and carceral measures. I conclude with thoughts about the emancipatory potential of queer and trans madness and a call to those invested in social justice for 2SLGBTQ people to interrogate the biomedical model of mental illness beyond the depathologization of gender and sexual dissidence.

© The Author(s), under exclusive license to Springer Nature
Switzerland AG 2022
M. D. Pilling, *Queer and Trans Madness*,
https://doi.org/10.1007/978-3-030-90413-5_6

Shifting the Paradigm: Allyship and Advocacy in Service Provision

As evidenced in Chapters 4 and 5, the mental health system often creates, contributes to, and increases mental distress. It is important to consider what needs to change within the system to minimize these harms because there continue to be many 2SLGBTQ people who want to use mental health services or who are forced do so through coercive means. In terms of thinking specifically about what needs to change within mental health service provision, many of the interviewees discussed the nature of their relationship to service providers and the necessity of shifting existing power dynamics within those relationships. This focus makes sense given that, as Mckeown et al. (2014) argue,

> it is often the relationships forged (or neglected) between workers and survivors that are at the heart of people's experiences of the mental health system—whether these experiences are profoundly positive or negative. Indeed, frontline workers are often seen as the bearers of a rightly maligned bio-psychiatry and, as such, often bear the brunt of survivors' critique. However, we think it is important to see workers as potential allies, not least because of the interdependency of workers' and survivors' interests and the fact that, often, both can feel alienated by their experience of the mental health system and, therefore, have a reciprocal interest in its democratic transformation. (p. 146)

While Mckeown et al. are referring mainly to formalized alliances between workers and survivors, such as trade unions, their points also apply to informal relationships. Alliances between workers and survivors are not easily achieved, given the shift in power inequities this would require. As the name suggests, the "helping professions" are predicated on a binary of helper/helped, and as Chapman and Withers (2019) state, "moving from helping/saving to working more mutually *with* can be conceptually difficult for people who have constructed their identities as helpers or allies" (p. 360; emphasis original). Chapman and Withers (2019) argue that part of making a shift in this dynamic is to think of allyship as "something you *do* rather than *who you are*" (p. 360; emphasis original).

This notion of allyship was discussed by some of the participants in explorations of positive experiences of service provision. For example, Charlotte,[1] a white, queer, cisgender woman stated:

> I think that mental health providers are super paternalistic and think that they know the right answer and the best thing for people and don't acknowledge context as much as they should be acknowledging context. I think they should be seeing their patients as allies and not as patients. I think that is a new kind of concept in healthcare where you don't have clients or patients. You have an ally and somebody that you work with to support.

A shift from envisioning people as patients to allies would mark a paradigm shift because of the implications about power relations. As Charlotte suggested, equitable power relations between practitioners and those experiencing mental distress would alter problematic paternalistic dynamics, as discussed in more detail in Chapter 4.

Likewise, Jacy, a Métis, trans, genderqueer person, was connected with a lesbian mental health worker and a gay youth and family development worker in Winnipeg as a teenager. These two workers helped him access social assistance and living arrangements. They also served as advocates for him within the mental health system. Jacy shared what happened with one of the workers after a particularly oppressive experience with a doctor:

> I told her about it and she was like, "That asshole." She's like, "I'm going down there right now." She opens her purse, applies her lipstick and takes off, went over to the clinic and fucking reamed them out. Like the doctor, the manager, she filed a formal complaint for me. It was amazing.

After this experience, Jacy never had trouble with that doctor again. This kind of advocacy is incredibly important. As a Métis, genderqueer youth navigating the child welfare system and the mental health system, Jacy experienced a lot of oppression. He felt that because these two workers were queer, they were motivated to help him and they were the ones he "talked to and connected with the most." He was still in touch with one of them as an adult and named her as "a really, really strong queer person in my life." This kind of advocacy is very different from medicating someone and sending them on their way and was far more helpful in aiding Jacy with addressing some of the conditions in his life that were creating distress. The need identified by the participants for service provision that treats people as allies would be supportive and provide advocacy that addresses social contexts. It stands in contrast to the realities described in Chapters 4 and 5.

Participants identified important aspects of allyship, including active listening skills, respect for agency and choice, and supportive counsel. Kylie, who identified as a white, queer, genderqueer person, said about her experiences with counsellors in Toronto: "They listen to you. They sit there and they listen to you and they don't really judge you, at least I don't think they do. If they do, they shut up [both laugh]. They do it privately." Similarly, Grace, a Korean, queer, gender-fluid woman, described her experiences with counsellors in Toronto as positive and very different from her experiences with psychiatrists:

> I've been fortunate to have really great counsellors who I've connected with and have challenged me, helped me unlearn things, and also really validated, which is the opposite of what I feel when I go see a psych. It's the opposite of validation. It's feeling like shit.

Displaying skills such as listening, respecting agency, and being supportive may seem like simple requirements, but the absence of them indicates the need for a paradigm shift in the way many practitioners currently operate.

Another aspect of allyship and advocacy is the importance of having a social justice approach to mental health service provision. This requires having knowledge of the ways in which power relations structure social inequities, processes of marginalization, and impacts of colonization, abuse, trauma, oppression, and violence. This goes beyond having a static understanding of culture and identities. As described in Chapters 4 and 5, many practitioners continue to pathologize 2SLGBTQ sexualities and gender identities. In order to combat these issues, some participants believed that practitioners needed to be aware of the history and ongoing practice of pathologizing 2SLGBTQ cultures and identities and how this impacts 2SLGBTQ people who experience mental distress. As one participant, Daxton, a white, French Canadian, queer, gay, cisgender man, told me, "gender and sexual identity that doesn't fit into the norms of society" have been considered mental illness and in some cases continue to be seen as such. He stated emphatically: "We can't operate in that way anymore and so I think there are definitely specific sensitivities required for a community that has for a long time been associated with mental illness in a really non-helpful way." Daxton believed that service providers becoming educated about this might make the mental health system more accessible to 2SLGBTQ people.

Many participants discussed the importance of service providers learning to place the focus on the effects of discrimination and oppression, rather than on sexuality, gender identity, and race. Collin, a white, gay, cisgender man, believed that service providers needed to be knowledgeable about the health impact of any kind of oppression. He discussed how service providers needed to take the effects of experiencing this kind of violence seriously. As he said: "I would say not just LGBTQ, I would also say anyone who's experiencing widespread hate I think would really be detrimental to your health to be told just for existing you're wrong and you're a terrible human being." Likewise, Owen, a Black, gay, cisgender man, emphasized that service providers needed to understand how "isolation and the shaming and the way people are conditioned to feel really uncomfortable in their own bodies requires more work to accept on the part of LGBTQ people." Owen stated that it was very important to accentuate that LGBTQ people don't "need more mental health resources because they're LGBTQ but because of the way they're made to be ashamed of themselves." Similarly, Silver, a mixed-race, queer, cisgender person, stated, regarding gender identity in particular, service providers needed to understand that "being transgender is not a mental illness and then in turn, there's nothing wrong with having a mental illness."

Many attributed the ability to use a critical approach to 2SLGBTQ mental distress to having experiential knowledge of marginalization. As one participant, Trevor, a white, queer, trans man, said, there is "very limited breadth of knowledge or experience" about race, class, sexuality, and gender among practitioners. However, this problem was not easily solved. As he said: "I don't know if you could read an extra chapter on queer stuff and then suddenly be the greatest doctor ever." For Trevor, understanding was achieved through experience: "I think it's experiential in a lot of ways. Unless you are queer or have a queer family member, been in proximity to it over a great length of time, then you can't really relate."

Likewise, Jared, a white, omnisexual, trans man, found that a lack of "commonalities" between himself and the practitioners he had seen made the interactions "cold and distant" because the practitioners were not "personally relating to the person, or if they do it seems really fake because there's no real commonality that they necessarily share." Jared found that the efforts of service providers to relate to him were not only fake but sometimes "offensive" because "the examples that they're drawing on are so radically simplistic compared to what I'm talking about." Jared had never encountered a service provider who shared key commonalities with him but believed that if he would encounter such a service provider, their interaction would be positive.

Some participants of colour discussed the importance of seeing service providers of colour. Sean, an East Asian, queer, trans man, said that he was helped by seeing a racialized counsellor who was "really good with the race issue." He found that when he discussed race and racism with white counsellors, he did not feel understood and stopped sharing these experiences. Similarly, Ameena, a South Asian, queer, cisgender woman, told me that "the biggest thing" was race because "that's the thing they see." She also considered disability an important factor and believed that seeing a racialized, disabled counsellor may have made a positive difference in her counselling experience because "possibly people [counsellors] wouldn't be so quick to make assumptions based on that [race and disability]." She acknowledged that this was "not necessarily true" but hoped it was.

This desire for service providers who shared commonalities in terms of social location can be seen as essentialist. Social difference is defined across a number of intersecting fronts, including but not limited to age, sexuality, gender, race, class, and disability, and none of these are static, fixed categories that share essential commonalities (Valentine, 2002). There is no guarantee that 2SLGBTQ practitioners will have anti-racist, anti-oppressive perspectives or share commonalities with 2SLGBTQ people seeking services. While lived experience is often the catalyst that leads people to learn social justice perspectives, it is possible to develop a critical consciousness through education without life experience of marginalization.

However, it is important to understand some participants' preference for practitioners who they perceived to be similarly socially located within the larger context of oppression in the health care system. As discussed in detail in Chapters 4 and 5, many service providers do not have a critical consciousness and continue to pathologize people on the basis of gender, sexuality, and race. In this context it is understandable that participants thought that practitioners with lived experience of marginalization would be better informed than those who did not. Additionally, perceived social location affects relationships between providers and those seeking services and often has an impact on trust. One of the cumulative impacts of experiencing oppression at the hands of health care practitioners was that some participants were less likely to trust practitioners they perceived as having privilege based on their social locations. For example, Silver, a mixed-race, queer, cisgender person, said that it "means a lot" for her to be able to discuss her "problems" with "someone who isn't straight" because if she is unsure of their sexuality she does not feel comfortable sharing her experiences. When I asked her to elaborate on the reasons for this, she told me that heterosexual practitioners are likely to make heterosexist assumptions and be unable to "relate" and "get it." Likewise, Dana, a white, Portuguese, French Canadian, lesbian, queer person, did not feel comfortable with her male counsellor: "I just didn't feel that he could connect with me. The lesbian issues are not the same as straight man issues."

As the participants' comments indicate, there is a need for more access to 2SLGBTQ practitioners and practitioners with a critical consciousness, along with practitioners who have experiential knowledge of oppression and marginalization and who incorporate a social justice approach to their service provision.

Shifting the Paradigm Requires Structural Change

As I have argued throughout this book, the harms produced by the mental health system are not the result of a few "bad" individual practitioners. There are systemic problems. Taking this seriously requires shifting the focus from individuals to structures. As Jacobson et al. (2010) state, "recovery should focus more on addressing social inequities and changing systems of mental health services and supports and less on changing the individuals who use these services and supports" (p. 13). This structural focus must reconfigure responses to mental distress using a broad lens that expands beyond the mental health system. As Weisser et al. (2011) argue, "mental health recovery services" should "include social supports such as housing, income security, employment options, accessible transit systems, paid parental leave, language classes, and educational opportunities" (p. 26). Likewise, Harper and Speed (2012) contend that more attention should be paid to identifying the "structural facilitators of recovery" such as "stable income, good housing, [and] employment" (p. 22). As this suggests, responses to mental distress need to be conceptualized in broad structural terms. Some have also suggested that a truth and reconciliation process may be necessary to begin healing the damage caused by mental health systems and to truly transform them (Spandler & McKeown, 2017).

While the changes outlined by participants thus far may seem focused on individuals, much of what they discussed is connected to broad structural change. For example, the types of positive experiences participants described in terms of practitioners who practiced allyship and advocacy were much more likely to be found within community health settings and in private practice with mental health counsellors rather than with psychiatrists. This indicates a strong need to expand publicly funded services so that people can freely access the kind of counselling and therapy that works for them, including that which addresses the impact of trauma and structural violence. There are large disparities in types of services and employment benefits that can be accessed based on income level (Ross et al., 2018). Further, the changes described by participants indicate the types of knowledge that need to be conveyed in the training of practitioners in all kinds in publicly funded settings. As the participants' comments demonstrate, this training must go beyond a cultural competence approach that reifies identities and cultural differences and focus instead on social justice approaches to allyship and advocacy by service providers.

As discussed in detail in Chapter 4, there is also a clear need for developing alternatives to the ways in which psychiatric medications are currently conceptualized and dispensed, that is, using a drug-centred approach (Moncrieff et al., 2013). It is necessary to support choice and agency in decision making regarding psychiatric drugs, including withdrawal support for those who decide to stop taking them. True choice and informed decision making requires more transparency in terms of the long-term outcomes and impact of all psychiatric drugs, which necessitates research and prescribing practices that are free from the influence of pharmaceutical companies. Additionally, Chapter 5 points to the need to address institutional policies and practices within psychiatric hospitals that cause the violence of misgendering to flourish, and, as discussed further below, an end to pathologizing and coercive, carceral practices.

De-Medicalized, Non-Carceral, Non-State Interventionist Responses to Queer and Trans Madness

While the changes outlined thus far are important and necessary, I cannot help but think, *it's not enough*. As I argued in Chapter 5, the charts from study two indicate that institutionalized trans and non-binary people experienced the compounded effects of structural inequities and interlocking systems of power and domination such as colonialism, white supremacy, and cisnormativity. The effects of these larger power dynamics were individualized by the psychiatric institution, and in some cases, responded to with punitive or coercive measures. These power structures are also deeply embedded within the institution and how it operates (see also Daley & Pilling, 2021). As I performed the data analysis for Chapter 5, I spent hours engaging with hundreds of pages of chart documentation on trans and non-binary people. It is perhaps impossible to convey the full extent of the dehumanization, violence, sadness, and distress that haunts these charts. Reading them felt like watching trans and non-binary community members drown, surrounded by people who were adding bricks to their load while smiling and claiming the extra weight would be helpful. Implementing the changes outlined thus far might feel like removing one or two of those bricks. It is important to do, but in the end, they are still going to sink.

The work that is compelling in terms of shifting large power structures and envisioning different futures is that of activists and scholars working in the overlapping areas of community care, community accountability, mutual aid, abolition, Disability Justice, Transformative Justice, and what has been referred to by some as mad/crip of colour critique (Ben-Moshe, 2020; Kim, 2017; Kim & Schalk, 2021). Most of this work is created and led by feminists of colour and/or trans and queer people, and/or disabled and mad Black, Indigenous, and people of colour (BIPOC) who work against the mutually constitutive forces of white supremacy, colonialism, ableism, sanism, transphobia, misogyny, homophobia, and heteropatriarchy (Ben-Moshe, 2020; Ben-Moshe et al., 2014; Berne, 2015; Clare, 2017; Daley & Radford, 2018; Davis, 2003; Dixon & Piepzna-Samarasinha, 2020; INCITE!, 2017; Piepzna-Samarasinha, 2018; Richie, 2005; Schenwar & Law, 2020; Smith & Stanley, 2015; Spade, 2020; Stanley & Spade, 2012; Vitulli, 2013). I do not purport to do justice to these large and complex bodies of work, in the following pages. Instead, I draw on some of the ideas that underpin this work to frame participants' narratives about strategies they employed to respond to madness, outside of the mental health system. I also provide recent examples of somewhat more formalized efforts to implement such strategies on a (relatively) larger scale. This is not to suggest that the responsibility for support should be placed exclusively on 2SLGBTQ communities; nor do I argue that such communities are utopian spaces free of problems. Rather, this discussion aims to explore the perspectives of queer and trans people with lived experience regarding the knowledge that already exists within communities (and is often discounted) about mutual aid and collective care in an effort to imagine de-medicalized, non-state interventionist, non-carceral approaches.

The Radical Potential of Collective Care and Mutual Aid

Though participants did not use the words mutual aid, they discussed what could be described as such. Dean Spade (2020) defines mutual aid as "collective coordination to meet each other's needs, usually from an awareness that the systems we have in place are not going to meet them. Those systems, in fact, have often created the crisis, or are making things worse" (p. 7). As a form of "reciprocal exchange for mutual benefit," mutual aid is built on a "model of solidarity not charity" that breaks down the binary of helper/helped by challenging the notion of "moral superiority of the giver over the receiver" (Piepzna-Samarasinha, 2018, p. 41). Mutual aid and collective care have recently received attention in mainstream (whitestream) circles. However, these practices have deep roots in Black, Indigenous, and Brown communities (Piepzna-Samarasinha, 2018; Spade, 2020). Mutual aid challenges the interlocking logics of capitalism, individualism, and independence that underpin mainstream (whitestream) notions of care. As Eales and Peers (2020) argue, the concept of care has long been used euphemistically to describe what is in fact state violence against "Indigenous, racialized, queer, disabled, and Mad folks" such as eugenics and institutionalization:

> The violences experienced under the guise of people being *cared about* and *cared for* and *taken into care* are just a few of the reasons that many disabled and Mad activists have, since the 1960s, started to renegotiate, if not reject, the term(s of) care. (p. 10; emphasis original)

Participants in both Toronto and Winnipeg were involved in what could be called community care and mutual aid as part of addressing mental distress, though this took different forms in each city. Toronto's large size and diverse population offered more opportunities for creating various kinds of communities. Toronto is unique in this respect among Canadian cities; even large cities like Vancouver do not compare. For example, one participant, Trevor, a white, queer, trans man, moved to Toronto from Vancouver and found that the social landscape was quite different:

When I first moved here I started hanging out with a lot of trans guys, because that was also new. I didn't hang out with as many trans guys before because there just wasn't as many; there was three or four of us. But now here [in Toronto] it's like you can meet ten right away and then there's ten other guys who hate those ten guys [laughs]. Like there's just so many more people.

As Trevor's comments indicate, the sheer number of people in Toronto made it more possible to create communities based on identities, behaviours, and experiences (such as being trans) for groups that are often marginalized within mainstream gay and lesbian communities. For many participants, this was a crucial part of addressing mental distress. For example, Grace, a Korean, queer, gender-fluid woman, discussed connections to Toronto communities that were "more open to certain differences," such as the "BDSM kink community" and the "poly community," as an important part of dealing with mental distress. As she said, "I can talk freely about my mental health stuff. And I use that as part of addressing some mental health things I'm going through." Likewise, Jared, a white, omnisexual, trans man, named the Toronto "BDSM leather community" as a place where people can deal with "deep problems":

People will have problems, like deep problems that they need to work out and live through and they have tactics for dealing with them that are definitely not within how you're supposed to deal with your issues. So I think that community is most aware of the diversity of people. So they don't expect everybody to be the same.

Jared also named the Toronto HIV/AIDS community as a supportive place to deal with mental distress:

Similar to BDSM and leather, people are more real and deep when they're in a safe environment. In the sense that if you're in a room with people that all know that they can trust each other, people will go a lot further. Those rooms are very valuable.

Creating kinship ties through community is especially salient for mad 2SLGBTQ people because the state and the nuclear family have been "the two sources disabled and sick people have most often been forced to rely on for care," and are often marked by "abuse and lack of control" (Piepzna-Samarasinha, 2018, p. 33). As Carter, a white, queer, trans man in Toronto, said:

> I think it's still pretty common as queer and trans people that we don't have the support from our families of origin that we need. And so creating those things is a pretty big part of what I want my community to be.

Likewise Kylie, a white, queer, genderqueer person, had a group of friends who served as a source of community care:

> I have friends who are consumers of the psychiatric system and we do create a small community for ourselves where we can talk about this stuff, we can be open about it and it's not stigmatizing. And we do support each other. There's maybe three or four of us, but it's one way that we can feel like we're supporting each other and we get it, because most of us are queer.

Shared experience of mental distress and being queer allowed for a valuable form of support for Kylie and her friends. Similarly, Sean, an East Asian, queer, trans man, was part of a group of queer and trans people who met regularly to discuss community accountability. This group was interested in figuring out a way to do "collective care" regarding mental health, which he described as follows:

> I feel like mental health is not really talked about as much, but in the community accountability group we are talking about it a lot. We're talking about disability, collective care, which is kind of new to me but I think it's an amazing concept, and a lot of people talk about things that they need to do for themselves, plus what they do if they need to outreach the community with collective care.

Sean was excited to encounter collective care as a way of addressing mental distress on a community level. Similarly, Carter, a white, queer, trans man, discussed being part of a "care collective" for "people with depression or who are going through grief" and noted that this was a "community that's created around being support systems for people." As Sean's and Carter's stories show, there were groups within Toronto 2SLGBTQ communities that were interested in radically reconfiguring support for mental distress as community care and mutual aid.

Some participants, like Owen, a Black, gay, cisgender man, found spaces of collective care through 2SLGBTQ organizations and groups. His involvement in a 2SLGBTQ student group offered "validation" and "a space where I could not constantly be questioned and made to feel like I'm strange or fucked up." Likewise, Logan, a biracial, queer, genderqueer person, found that participating in a trans-focused peer support group run by a community centre fostered a connection with one of the facilitators, who "checks up" on him regarding "mental health" and "disability."

Many participants in Winnipeg also named communities as places of support and as vital in addressing mental distress, sometimes directly challenging mainstream notions of care. For example, Chase, a white, gay, cisgender man, challenged the notion of individualism, stating that the idea that "everyone's responsible for their own mental health is too much along the same lines of the rugged individual surviving in the wilderness." Chase believed that this was not an accurate depiction of "how people function, as social creatures" given that they are interdependent. For Chase this meant that "there really needs to be less of an institutionalization of mental health and more of a grassroots community focus."

Many participants identified isolation as a factor that created and exacerbated mental distress, while they saw connection with community as an antidote. For example, Levi, a white, Jewish, gay, cisgender man in Winnipeg, said:

I think when people are isolated, that's the worst possible thing. If we're gonna talk mental health, isolation is one of the key issues. Whether you're isolated socially, medically, whatever, when you're on your own and you don't feel connected up, you're gonna get sick.

The small size of Winnipeg queer and trans communities had positive effects in terms of making connections and creating support. Many felt that the small size made it more conducive to finding community through friends. Nova, a Métis, lesbian, cisgender woman, told me that the Winnipeg community is "so small that it's more like one on one." For her, this provided the opportunity to connect with other 2SLGBTQ people who experienced mental distress. She said: "You know who has mental health issues. Maybe not everybody, but you start to know some people." For some, like Nova, the smallness allowed for making connections. Likewise, Cami, a white, queer, person, found that seeing the same people over the course of many years in the queer community meant that she eventually came to know others who experienced mental distress through talking more "deeply" with people in the community. This allowed her to create a supportive community of queer friends who also experienced distress and rejected medical methods of addressing it:

It provides a basis of support for people. I'm also a manic depressive, up and down all over the board. And for the group of people that were having the same types of things going on, there's certainly a support in that because you can recognize what's going on and you can recognize what's happening in your drug cycle. It's an odd community support system but it works. Because your friend would see what was going on, and instead of taking you to the doctor or to wherever you'd get a shot, you'd do some drugs and you'd be fine.

For Cami and her friends, taking drugs that were deemed recreational instead of psychiatric was part of addressing her mental distress. Doing this with a group of friends offered a way of monitoring her moods and considering how the drugs were affecting her.

Intra-Community Oppression in Toronto and Winnipeg

As the participant narratives demonstrate, creating and participating in mutual aid and collective care played a crucial role in addressing mental distress. However, the creation of such communities was hard-won, and the communities remained marginalized in both cities. Many participants referred to mainstream queer communities where various kinds of oppression ran rampant, leaving them feeling isolated. For example, Owen, a Black, gay, cisgender man, described staying quiet about his attraction to "chubby men" because fatphobia meant people were more "freaked out" by his attraction to fat bodies than by his attraction to men.

In addition to fatphobia, many named the prevalence of racism, ableism, and classism as exclusionary forces within 2SLGBTQ communities. In Toronto, Silver, a mixed-race, queer, cisgender person, described this as follows:

> The mainstream queer spaces tend to be super, super white. And it's the kind of thing that I used to be more comfortable with but not anymore. So it's like, okay I could go but none of the other queer people I know would feel welcome. With disability stuff once again, like, why is everyone white? Or there's an awful lot of straight people, and so on. So it's hard to find people that I have a lot of stuff in common with, identity wise.

Silver also described a lack of interest within mainstream queer communities in making events accessible and a lack of acknowledgment that "disability intersects with poverty." Similarly, Ameena, a South Asian, queer, cisgender woman, described an event that was advertised as being created by and for disabled queer people but was "really exclusionary" because it was "such a mainstream kind of queer," not physically accessible, and featured an MC who made ableist and racist jokes, such as making fun of a performer with a "non-Anglo name." For Ameena, experiencing this kind of event meant that she felt isolated and no longer sought out community:

> The worst part was that I was hoping and looking forward to some kind of community space, and it was just such a huge disappointment. Another reason why I avoid getting into these kinds of spaces, because of shit like this. It's just such a huge, crushing disappointment.

Ameena's story highlights the importance of a supportive, anti-oppressive community by illuminating the impact of experiencing the opposite. Likewise, Grace described being asked to stop attending meetings of a community of women of colour based on her physical and mental health. She was unable to attend some meetings because of her physical health and was sometimes "checked out" when she was present because of her mental health. Grace was deeply hurt by the ableist and sanist request to leave the community: "I'm still really, really struggling, like not a day goes by that it's not painful." As these stories show, creating community that was inclusive and anti-oppressive in every respect was an ongoing struggle in Toronto.

This was also a challenge in Winnipeg. Winnipeg is the largest city in Manitoba and at the time of interviewing, it was larger than the second largest city, Brandon, by approximately 68,000 people. This makes Winnipeg, at 700,000 people, a big city, but on a much smaller scale than Toronto. The small size of the Winnipeg 2SLGBTQ community meant that there were fewer anti-oppressive community spaces and events. There were fewer opportunities for what Jacy, a Métis, trans, genderqueer person, called "radical queer community." As he also pointed out, much of the Winnipeg 2SLGBTQ community is a bar-based culture:

> The main queer community is really the bar scene, especially in Winnipeg. In bigger cities you definitely have more options, but in Winnipeg it's pretty small. There's not like a radical queer community. It's mostly just the bar scene and then friends. So I have friends. But I've never really felt a part of any queer kind of scene or whatever.

Bars are generally inaccessible spaces for many reasons, including the importance of alcohol, physical inaccessibility, and daunting conditions (like crowds of people and loud music) that can be difficult to navigate for some who experience mental distress. As Jacy pointed out, bar culture was not amenable to radical queer community where alternative forms of support could be organized, such as the collective care arrangements described by Toronto participants.

Racism also made some Winnipeg LGBTQ community spaces hostile places for BIPOC participants. At the time of interviewing, there were two queer bars in Winnipeg, Gio's and Club 200. As Dylan, a Métis, queer, cisgender man, told me, these bars had "very, very different clientele":

> I don't think a lot of the clientele [from Club 200] would feel comfortable or even be allowed to get into Gio's, because a lot of the clientele from Club 200 is primarily Aboriginal, two-spirited, some trans folks. Whereas Gio's is much more non-Aboriginal. I've heard people talk about it in the community, right. I've heard people be like, "I'm not going to Club 200. There's too many Indians there."

As Dylan pointed out, racism directed at Indigenous people created exclusionary and racist social spaces. Another participant, Cheyenne, a Métis, bi-queer, cisgender woman, told me that "community celebrations" that took place at Gio's were often avoided by BIPOC because they were "very centred around white privilege." Cheyenne gave an example of a drag event that she described as "Pocahontas, John Smith fucking pow wow party shit." The organizers defended this racist, anti-Indigenous event on the basis of having included an Indigenous drag performer who was apparently "fine with it." Cheyenne was angry that the organizers used this tokenistic defense. She said that many people in the community were oblivious to how racist these kinds of events were and that "the only people who are aware of how weird it is to have that kind of celebration are the people of colour who avoid it." As Dylan and Cheyenne suggested, two-spirit and Indigenous LGBTQ people experience racism within LGBTQ communities, making some community spaces sources of oppression rather than support. However, their comments also suggest that Club 200 provided a more supportive place for two-spirit and Indigenous LGBTQ people, though this was not stated directly by any of the participants.

As this discussion shows, many participants in both Toronto and Winnipeg believed in the importance of mutual aid and community care as crucial components of responding to mental distress. Community building in both cities was complicated and often fraught with tensions regarding intra-community oppression. However, it was clear that connection with others and support from people who had similar experiences were key in addressing mental distress. Communities that have been marginalized or targeted by the state often have knowledge and practices of collective survival survival that reject coercive and oppressive tactics employed within service provision and medical treatments. As Coles et al. (2013) state, "freeing ourselves from established conventions of ideals, actions and professional customs can leave people feeling anxious and uncertain in how to make sense of madness, and how to help and offer support" (p. xii). Participants' stories about mutual aid and community building offer one way to begin an exploration of de-medicalized, non-carceral, non-state interventionist ways of responding to mental distress. In what comes next, I discuss how the stakes of such exploration are heightened in cases of suicidality and crisis.

Responding to Crisis: Resisting Coercion and Carcerality

It is imperative to think critically about crisis response because crises such as acute suicidality and heightened states of distress often compel even those who critique and resist carceral, coercive, and state-interventionist means of responding to mental distress to employ these methods because we do not know what else to do. When we or a loved one is in crisis we might consider relying on the carceral state in some way, usually by involving a psychiatric facility or by calling the police. Why is this a problem? As has been demonstrated by the devastating consequences of wellness checks conducted by the police,[2] a call to 911 can end in the murder of those in distress at the hands of police, especially those who are Black, Indigenous or a person of colour. This is sometimes imagined (often by white Canadians) to be an American problem. However, the deaths of Andrew Loku, Regis Korchinski-Paquet, Eliza Choudry, and D'Andre Campbell indicate that the deadly combination of systemic sanism and racism thrives in Canadian law enforcement too (for a discussion of anti-Black sanism in particular, see Abdillahi et al. [2017] and Meerai et al. [2016]). Mad trans and non-binary people, particularly those who are BIPOC, are also at high risk of violence from police. For example, the conditions under which a Black, trans woman died after Toronto police took her into custody under Ontario's Mental Health Act are still unknown, and she was misgendered in communications by the agency responsible for overseeing police (Ontario's Special Investigation's Unit) (Nasser, 2020). A national study of trans and non-binary people in Canada found that 73% of racialized trans and non-binary people and 50% of white trans and non-binary people "worried about being stopped or harassed by police or security because of who they are" (Chih et al., 2020, p. 8). Thirty-three per cent of racialized respondents had refrained from calling police in the past five years, with 24% refraining from calling 911 for emergency medical attention (Chih et al., 2020). The mental health system is also implicated in these issues. In Ontario, people experiencing mental distress can be apprehended by the police under the Mental Health Act as an emotionally disturbed person and taken to a psychiatric ward/institution where they can be held involuntarily for up to 72 hours for psychiatric assessment.[3]

Recent calls to defund the police have sometimes been accompanied by demands to replace police officers with social workers in 911 emergency responses to mental health crises. At first glance, this may seem unproblematic or at least highly preferable to unleashing the police on people in distress. However, these calls underestimate the harms that can be inflicted by social work (see Chapman & Withers, 2019), the mental health system, psychiatry, and the carceral logics that underpin them. As Kaufman-Mthimkhulu (2020) argues, those who have never been institutionalized in a psychiatric ward/hospital may envision them as places of "healing and treatment" for BIPOC (and, I would add, trans and non-binary people) rather than of violence and trauma (para 2). Kaufman-Mthimkhulu states, "psychiatric institutions are...part of the carceral state. This means that they are part of the many systems that function to contain people, take away their locus of control, offer surveillance, isolate them from their communities, and limit their freedom" (para 2). As she goes on to argue, "as it stands now, if we tried to replace cops with social workers, we would be trading in one system of policing for a different system of policing" (para 8). Likewise, Ben-Moshe refers to the practice of replacing police with social workers as "weaponizing social work" (The New Press, 2021). This practice is an example of what she calls carceral sanism, a form "of carcerality that contribute[s] to the oppression of mad or mentally ill populations under the guise of treatment" (Ben-Moshe, 2020, p. 58). Calls to defund the police must include analyses of the interlocking nature of sanism, anti-Blackness, and other forms of racism, colonialism, as well as the transphobia and cisnormativity, that position trans, non-binary, and gender nonconforming people as abject and abnormal and, therefore, at risk of violence at the hands of police and mental health practitioners.

What then, can we do when confronted with acute distress and suicidality? In what follows I highlight a handful of initiatives that are de-medicalized, non-carceral, and non-state interventionist responses to acute distress. I devote space to these initiatives because it is so hard to imagine possibilities beyond the biomedical model and because of the pressing nature of imagining and creating responses that are free of carceral logics and coercion, and that honour bodily autonomy and interdependence. I chose initiatives that focus on crisis response and trans and queer people, and initiatives with an explicit intersectional or anti-racist framework foregrounding the mutually constitutive nature of racism and sanism. While it is difficult to find initiatives with these explicit foci, my account should not be seen as exhaustive in terms of de-medicalized, non-state interventionist, and non-carceral responses to mental distress and crisis. There is a long history of mad organizing that has created de-medicalized, non-carceral responses to madness (see, for example, the Fireweed Collective [formerly The Icarus Project], Inner Compass Initiative, Leeds Survivor Led Crisis Service, Live & Learn Inc.'s site peerrespite.com, models based on Diabasis house and Soteria houses, and many others). There is also a long history of anti-racist, social justice, and abolitionist organizing that has created numerous initiatives that intersect with or address crisis from a de-carceral perspective. For more information, I direct readers to the edited collection *Beyond Survival: Strategies and Stories from the Transformative Justice Movement* (Dixon & Piepzna-Samarasinha, 2020) as well as lists on Elliot Fukui's website www.madque er.org and Liat Ben-Moshe's website www.liatbenmoshe.com/resources.

Trans Lifeline

Founded in 2014, Trans Lifeline is a national hotline in the United States and Canada that was created in response to the very high rates of suicide in trans communities. They self-describe as "radical community care" that "provides trans peer support that's been divested from police since day one" (translifeline.org). Unlike most suicide hotlines, Trans Lifeline does not endorse "non-consensual active rescue." In other words, they do not call emergency responders unless requested to by a caller. As they state, "over and over again, we hear from our community…that one of the main deciding factors in whether they reach out for help is whether they will have to deal with active rescue" (Trans Lifeline, 2020, p. 136). Based on a survey they conducted, they found that non-consensual active rescue can increase suicidality for trans community members. This is due to a number of factors, including the discrimination trans and non-binary people experience at the hands of police as well as in mental health settings (Trans Lifeline, 2020). Based on the principles of mutual aid, Trans Lifeline also distributes microgrants to trans people for the purposes of changing names and gender markers on identification, reserving 75% of these funds for BIPOC. In doing so, Trans Lifeline recognizes the additional barriers faced by BIPOC because of white supremacy. They also distribute microgrants to trans people who were incarcerated and recently released, for commissary, changes to identification, and re-entry. Trans Lifeline employs an "abolitionist framework that pre-empts crises by connecting trans people with each other , because the most powerful tool we have for safety is each other" (https://translifeline.org/about/#princples).

Suicide Intervention for Weirdos, Freaks, and Queers (Carly Boyce)

Suicide Intervention for Weirdos, Freaks, and Queers is a workshop that was developed by Carly Boyce in Toronto, Ontario, in 2016. This workshop employs "peer and community-based strategies for supporting folks in our lives who might be suicidal, as well as examining the beliefs and structures that keep suicide conversations under wraps" (Boyce, n.d.). In a zine based on the workshop, Boyce writes that a motivating factor in creating the workshop was to create space for discussions with those who do not want to involve police or who are supporting people who have experienced harm in psychiatric settings about how to provide support. Boyce articulates an intersectional analysis that considers the ways in which multiple interlocking systems of oppression shape who wants to die by suicide and who has access to support. The zine and a webinar of the same name are both accessible at www.tinylantern.net.

Mad Queer Organizing Strategies (Elliott Fukui)

Based in California, Mad Queer Organizing Strategies is the work of Elliott Fukui. Since 2018, Fukui has been offering resources and trainings to build capacity for collective care, based in the principles of mutual aid, Disability Justice, and abolition. Fukui's resources focus on a range of topics, including "wellness and safety planning for emotional crisis to using maps to engage with the personal and political impacts of trauma" with the goal of "remind[ing] people that our greatest and most invaluable resource in the struggle for liberation is each other" (Fukui, n.d.). Fukui also offers a workbook entitled Surviving the Apocalypse Together: A Mutual Aid Safety and Wellness Planning for COVID-19, which is available on Fukui's website www.madqueer.org.

Project LETS

Founded and led by Stefanie Kaufman-Mthimkhulu, Project LETS is a national, grassroots organization in the United States that builds "transformative peer support collectives and community mental health care structures that do not depend on state-sanctioned systems that trap our folks in the medical/prison-industrial complex" (Project LETS, n.d.). Project LETS does not focus specifically on queer and trans people but espouses an anti-oppression framework as well as the principles of mutual aid, peer support, Disability Justice, and abolition. It offers a number of programmes and services, including peer support in post-secondary contexts. Project LETS is developing this programme for the community context in order to replace police in responses to mental distress calls (Kaufman-Mthimkhulu, 2020). It also offers training and workshops in crisis response, anti-racist solidarity, carceral ableism, and suicide as a political issue.

In many ways, all of these initiatives hold similar values to those expressed by the interviewees regarding mutual aid and collective care. These initiatives value community knowledge in that they are created by and for the people they serve and are grounded in communities' actual needs. They are aimed at increasing the capacity of communities to respond to crisis without relying on the police or psychiatric institutions/wards. They acknowledge the existence and impact of interlocking and mutually constitutive systems of power and oppression and seek to redress these harms wherever possible. Distress is positioned as an understandable response to life events, and the behaviours that manifest in response to such circumstances have meaning. People experiencing distress are treated as agents in their own right who are making decisions that make sense within the context of their lives. In many ways these initiatives create space for existing in ways that fall outside the norm—as queer, trans, and mad. This stands in sharp contrast to the medical approaches described throughout this book. In describing these initiatives, I do not mean to be prescriptive about crisis response or to suggest that the responsibility of care should fall exclusively to queer, trans, and other oppressed communities or that the cost and responsibility for them be downloaded onto individuals in neoliberal ways that sidestep state accountability. Rather, these initiatives provide inspiration for the ways we could reimagine support and crisis response and are evidence of the ways in which this is already being done. They are examples of initiatives that are "breaking down things that oppress and building up things that nourish" (Bassichis et al., 2011, p. 37). There are multiple avenues towards a world in which mad, queer, and trans people experience true care and support. As Piepzna-Samarasinha (2018) writes,

> I want us to dream mutual aid in our post apocalyptic revolutionary societies where everyone gets to access many kinds of care—from friends and internet strangers, from disabled community centres, and from some kind of non-fucked-up non-state state that would pay caregivers well and give them health benefits and time off and enshrine sick and disabled autonomy and choice. I want us to keep dreaming and experimenting with all these big, ambitious ways we dream care for each other into being. (p. 65)

I began this chapter with a discussion of participants' ideas about what they would like to see changed within the mental health system, including shifts in power inequities between practitioners and those who use their services, and workers who employ a social justice perspective and advocate for service users. I also outlined some necessary structural changes based on arguments established in Chapters 4 and 5. While these changes are important, it could be said that there is not much about them that is truly liberatory. In fact, it is possible that some of the changes discussed, while necessary, may make problematic services more palatable, increasing support for these approaches even within queer and trans communities.[4] In the second half of this chapter, I focused on participant narratives about mutual aid and collective care within queer and trans communities. I discussed some of the problems with carceral and state-interventionist responses to acute distress and suicidality and described some recent initiatives that offer other ways to respond.

It is my hope that this book will contribute to conversations that are already happening in various activist and scholarly circles about de-medicalized, non-carceral approaches to understanding and responding to mental distress. Given the longstanding and ongoing relationship between ideas about mental pathology, gender and sexual dissidence, and race, these are issues of great importance to 2SLGBTQ people and BIPOC.[5] As I have argued throughout this book, it is necessary to broaden the critique of the biomedical model of mental illness beyond the diagnoses that refer explicitly to gender and sexual dissidence and to be cautious about advocating for more access to treatment without critically examining what constitutes treatment and the impact of medicalized strategies, including carceral and coercive tactics, on mad 2SLGBTQ people. As I have shown, further incorporating queer and trans people into mental health systems can run counter to the desired goal of improving health and may in fact result in iatrogenic harm and punitive, oppressive responses to distress. Participant narratives regarding their experiences with mental health care practitioners demonstrate the limitations of medical strategies to address mental distress, especially given the vexed context in which this occurs for 2SLGBTQ people and BIPOC. Chart documentation of trans and non-binary patients shows that mental health care practitioners do not make objective assessments of mental health and illness; rather, the process is enculturated and reflects oppressive sociocultural values. A critical analysis of the charts provided empirical evidence for the claim that trans and non-binary people's survival strategies and resistance to transphobia and oppression are individualized and psychiatrized.

As this final chapter has shown, there are other ways of understanding and responding to distress. De-medicalized and non-coercive ways of understanding and responding to distress and crisis have deep roots in mad, queer, trans, and BIPOC communities, and offer a way forward, away from the psy complex. This can be seen in community knowledge about how to take care of one another, in kinship ties outside of the nuclear family, in the centring of the most marginalized, in the redistribution of wealth, and, in some cases, the refusal to be assimilated and disciplined into cisnormative, medicalized understandings of our identities, ways of being, experiences, and bodies. This is the emancipatory promise of queer and trans madness.

Notes

1. All names are pseudonyms.
2. A wellness check is when police go to a person's home, usually in response to a 911 call regarding a person in distress. This can result in police violence against BIPOC. See, for example, https://www.aptnnews.ca/national-news/mountie-reassigned-after-video-shows-officer-entering-cree-mans-home-with-axe/.
3. After 72 hours has elapsed, a person can be held involuntarily under a certificate of involuntary admission (Form 3). See https://www.lhsc.on.ca/media/3109/download.
4. For more on this problem and a discussion of reformist versus abolitionist approaches in psychiatry, see Ben-Moshe (2020) and Burstow (2014).
5. These groups are obviously not mutually exclusive, but throughout this book I sometimes name BIPOC explicitly because due to white supremacy, it is often the case that when BIPOC are not explicitly named, it is because their experiences are erased.

References

Abdillahi, I., Meerai, S., & Poole, J. (2017). When the suffering is compounded: Towards anti-Black sanism. In S. Wehbi & H. Parada (Eds.), *Reimagining anti-oppression social work practice* (pp. 109–122). Canadian Scholars Press.

Bassichis, M., Lee, A., & Spade, D. (2011). Building an abolitionist trans and queer movement with everything we've got. In N. Smith & E. A. Stanley (Eds.), *Captive genders: Trans embodiment and the prison industrial complex* (pp. 15–40). AK Press.

Ben-Moshe, L. (2020). Decarcerating disability: Deinstitutionalization and prison abolition. *University of Minnesota Press*. https://doi.org/10.5749/j.ctv10vm2vw

Ben-Moshe, L., Chapman, C., & Carey, A. C. (2014). *Disability incarcerated: Imprisonment and disability in the United States and Canada*. Palgrave Macmillan. https://doi.org/10.1057/9781137388476

Berne, P. (2015). *Disability justice—A working draft by Patty Berne*. https://www.sinsinvalid.org/blog/disability-justice-a-working-draft-by-patty-berne

Boyce, C. (n.d.). *Suicide intervention resources for weirdos, freaks, and queers*. Tiny Lantern. Retrieved August 23, 2021, from https://www.tinylantern.net/suicide-intervention-resources

Burstow, B. (2014). The withering away of psychiatry: An attrition model for antipsychiatry. In B. Burstow, B. LeFrançois, & S. Diamond (Eds.), *Psychiatry disrupted: Theorizing resistance and crafting the (r)evolution* (pp. 34–51). McGill-Queen's University Press.

Chapman, C., & Withers, A. J. (2019). *Violent history of benevolence: Interlocking oppression in the moral economies of social working*. University of Toronto Press.

Chih, C., Wilson-Yang, Q., Dhaliwal, K., Khatoon, N., Redman, N., Malone, R., Islam, S., & Persad, Y. (2020). *Health and well-being among racialized trans and non-binary people in Canada*. Trans Pulse Canada. Retrieved August 23, 2021, from https://transpulsecanada.ca/results/report-health-and-well-being-among-racialized-trans-and-non-binary-people-in-canada/

Clare, E. (2017). *Brilliant imperfection: Grappling with cure*. Duke University Press.

Coles, S., Keenan, S., & Diamond, B. (2013). *Madness contested: Power and practice*. PCCS Books.

Daley, A., & Pilling, M. D. (2021). *Interrogating psychiatric narratives of madness: Documented lives*. Palgrave Macmillan.

Daley, A., & Radford, K. (2018). Queer and trans incarceration distress: Considerations from a mad queer abolitionist perspective. In A. Mills & K. Kendall (Eds.), *Mental health in prisons* (pp. 285–307). Palgrave Macmillan. https://doi.org/10.1007/978-3-319-94090-8_12

Davis, A. (2003). *Are prisons obsolete?* Seven Stories Press.

Dixon, E., & Piepzna-Samarasinha, L. L. (2020). *Beyond survival: Strategies and stories from the transformative justice movement*. AK Press.

Eales, L., & Peers, D. (2020). Care haunts, hurts, heals: The promiscuous poetics of queer crip Mad care. *Journal of Lesbian Studies, 25*(3), 1–19. https://doi.org/10.1080/10894160.2020.1778849

Fukui, E. (n.d.). *Building maps, strategies and processes for liberation: Mad Queer organizing strategies*. Retrieved August 23, 2021, from www.madqueer.org

Harper, D., & Speed, E. (2012). Uncovering recovery: The resistible rise of recovery and resilience. *Studies in Social Justice, 6*(1), 9–26. https://doi.org/10.26522/ssj.v6i1.1066

INCITE! Women of Colour Against Violence. (2017). *The revolution will not be funded: Beyond the non-profit industrial complex.* Duke University Press.

Jacobson, N., Farah, D., & Toronto Recovery and Cultural Diversity Community of Practice. (2010). *Recovery through the lens of cultural diversity.* Wellesley Institute. Retrieved August 23, 2021, from https://www.wellesleyinstitute.com/publications/recovery-through-the-lens-of-cultural-diversity-2010/

Kaufman-Mthimkhulu, S. L. (2020). *We don't need cops to become social workers: We need peer support + community response networks.* Stefanie Lyn Kaufman-Mthimkhulu. Retrieved August 23, 2021, from https://blog.usejournal.com/we-dont-need-cops-to-become-social-workers-we-need-peer-support-b8e6c4ffe87a

Kim, J. B. (2017). Toward a crip-of-color critique: Thinking with Minich's "enabling whom?" *Lateral, 6*, 1. https://doi.org/10.25158/L6.1.14

Kim, J. B., & Schalk, S. (2021). Reclaiming the radical politics of self-care: A crip-of-color critique. *South Atlantic Quarterly, 120*(2), 325–342. http://samischalk.com/wp-content/uploads/2021/05/Schalk_Black-Disability-Gone-Viral_CLA-Journal-2021.pdf

Mckeown, M., Cresswell, M., & Spandler, H. (2014). Deeply engaged relationships: Alliances between mental health workers and psychiatric survivors in the UK. In B. Burstow, B. A. LeFrançois, & S. Diamond (Eds.), *Psychiatry disrupted: Theorizing resistance and crafting the (r)evolution* (pp. 145–162). McGill-Queen's Press-MQUP.

Meerai, S., Abdillahi, I., & Poole, J. (2016). An introduction to anti-Black sanism. *Intersectionalities: A Global Journal of Social Work Analysis, Research, Polity, and Practice, 5*(3), 18–35. https://journals.library.mun.ca/ojs/index.php/IJ/article/view/1682

Moncrieff, J., Cohen, D., & Mason, J. (2013). The patient's dilemma: An analysis of users' experiences of taking neuroleptic drugs. In S. Coles, S. Keenan, & B. Diamond (Eds.), *Madness contested: Power and practice* (pp. 3–22). PCCS Books.

Nasser, S. (2020, November 3). Members of LGBTQ community demand answers after Black trans woman dies in police custody. *CBC News.*

Retrieved August 23, 2021, from https://www.cbc.ca/news/canada/toronto/black-trans-woman-crisis-toronto-siu-1.5787990

Piepzna-Samarasinha, L. L. (2018). *Care work: Dreaming disability justice.* Arsenal Pulp Press.

Project LETS. (n.d.). *Our mission. Project LETS.* Retrieved August 23, 2021, from https://projectlets.org/about

Richie, B. (2005). Queering antiprison work: African American lesbians in the juvenile justice system. In J. Sudbury (Ed.), *Global lockdown: Race, gender, and the prison-industrial complex* (pp. 73–85). Routledge.

Ross, L. E., Gibson, M. F., Daley, A., Steele, L. S., & Williams, C. C. (2018). In spite of the system: A qualitatively-driven mixed methods analysis of the mental health services experiences of LGBTQ people living in poverty in Ontario, Canada. *PloS One, 13*(8). https://doi.org/10.1371/journal.pone.0201437

Schenwar, M., & Law, V. (2020). *Prison by any other name: The harmful consequences of popular reforms.* The New Press.

Smith, N., & Stanley, E. A. (2015). *Captive genders: Trans embodiment and the prison industrial complex.* AK Press.

Spade, D. (2020). *Mutual aid: Building solidarity during this crisis (and the next).* Verso Books.

Spandler, H., & McKeown, M. (2017). Exploring the case for truth and reconciliation in mental health services. *Mental Health Review Journal, 22*(2), 83–94.

Stanley, E. A., & Spade, D. (2012). Queering prison abolition, now? *American Quarterly, 64*(1), 115–127. Retrieved August 21, 2021, from http://againstequality.org/files/queering_prison_abolition_now.pdf

Stewart, C. (2020, August 27). Mountie reassigned after video shows officer entering Cree man's home with axe. *APTN National News.* Retrieved August 23, 2021, from https://www.aptnnews.ca/national-news/mountie-reassigned-after-video-shows-officer-entering-cree-mans-home-with-axe/

The New Press. (2021, May 21). *Beyond alternatives: Disability, madness and prison abolition [webinar].* https://www.youtube.com/watch?v=CqaOgVzwCZ4

Trans Lifeline. (2020). Why no nonconsensual active rescue? In E. Dixon & L. L. Piepzna-Samarasinha (Eds.), *Beyond survival: Strategies and stories from the transformative justice movement* (pp. 135–140). AK Press.

Valentine, G. (2002). People like us: Negotiating sameness and difference in the research process. In P. Moss (Ed.), *Feminist geography in practice: Research and methods* (pp. 116–126). Wiley-Blackwell.

Vitulli, E. W. (2013). Queering the carceral: Intersecting queer/trans studies and critical prison studies. *GLQ: A Journal of Gay and Lesbian Studies, 19*(1), 111–123.

Weisser, J., Jamer, B., & Morrow, M. (2011). *A critical exploration of social inequities in the mental health recovery literature.* Centre for the Study of Gender, Social Inequities and Mental Health, Simon Fraser University. Retrieved August 23, 2021, from https://www.researchgate.net/profile/Marina-Morrow/publication/264877917_The_Recovery_Dialogues_A_Critical_Exploration_of_Social_Inequities_in_Mental_Health_Recovery/links/5a2d66e6aca2728e05e2e06e/The-Recovery-Dialogues-A-Critical-Exploration-of-Social-Inequities-in-Mental-Health-Recovery.pdf

Appendix

Methods: Queer and Trans Madness (Study One)

Chapters 3, 4, and 6 draw on data from a study entitled Mad Queers, Mad Trans People: Lived Experience at the Intersection of Gender, Sexuality, Race, Class, Dis/Ability and Mental Health, which for the purposes of this book I refer to as the Queer and Trans Madness study. Between 2010 and 2012, I conducted 37 qualitative interviews with queer and trans people about mental distress, identity, community, and experiences in the workplace and in healthcare settings. In this book, I focus on the data regarding mental distress, identity, community, and healthcare.[1]

Nineteen participants were recruited in Winnipeg, Manitoba, and 18 in Toronto, Ontario. I chose to interview in Winnipeg and Toronto in order to allow for the possibility of making comparative assessments and exploring the differences between living in a metropolis with a strong psychiatric survivor community and a smaller city with fewer community resources. Toronto, the biggest city in Canada, had a population of about 2.79 million and 5.5 million in the Greater Toronto Area at the time of interviewing. Toronto is much more heavily populated than Winnipeg,

M. D. Pilling, *Queer and Trans Madness*,
https://doi.org/10.1007/978-3-030-90413-5

the capital of Manitoba, which at the time of interviewing had a population of approximately 700,000. Yet the two are both "big cities" in that Winnipeg is the largest city in Manitoba and larger than the second biggest city, Brandon, by approximately 68,000 people. According to the 2011 census, Toronto had the largest number of residents who were immigrants, at 49% (Statistics Canada, 2013a). In comparison, 28% of Winnipeg residents and 21% of Canada's total population were immigrants (Statistics Canada, 2013b). Forty-nine per cent of Toronto residents identified as visible minorities as opposed to 21% in Winnipeg and 19% nationally (Statistics Canada, 2013a, 2013b). Notably, Indigenous peoples made up 0.8% of the total Toronto population at the time of interviewing, compared to 11% of Winnipeg's and 4.3% nationally (Statistics Canada, 2013a, 2013b). Winnipeg's larger Indigenous population made the intersections of sanism and other forms of oppression with colonial violence more visible in the interviews that took place in Winnipeg.

As these numbers show, Toronto is unusual in that it is home to significantly more immigrants and visible minorities than any other Canadian city. In this respect, Winnipeg is a more typical Canadian city, and including it as a research site allowed me to extend my analysis beyond Toronto. Further, as the province with the largest population and 21 universities, Ontario is often the site of Canadian research studies. Southwestern Ontario and Toronto in particular, with its large and diverse population, is a common choice for researchers. Adding a second, less researched site broadens the perspective and shows what commonalities exist, despite any provincial and local differences. Indeed, I found that there were far more similarities than differences in the participants' narratives, and these are emphasized throughout the book.

Qualitative Interviewing

When it came time to compose the call for participants, I struggled with what terminology to use in terms of mental health in order to reach the people I was interested in interviewing. When conceptualizing the project, I knew that I wanted to conduct interviews with those who self-identified as mad or mentally ill or who had been deemed as such (or, alternatively, psychiatric survivor, service user, consumer, or another term) and who also identified as lesbian, gay, bisexual, queer, trans, or another term. I say "deemed as such" as well as "self-identify" in order to indicate that I was interested in speaking with those who had a medical diagnosis concerning their mental health as well as those who did not, in order to avoid perpetuating the notion that medical authorities should be the ones to determine whether someone is mad. I was not interested in framing my sample in terms of how the participants had been diagnosed because this ascribed too much weight to medical categorization, and I wanted to capture a range of attitudes towards diagnosis and self-identification. For example, I anticipated that some participants would reject medical labels altogether, some would use them in certain contexts and not others, and others would fully embrace them. It was difficult to convey all of this in a succinct call for participants. The following excerpt from my call for participants illustrates how I approached this:

> There are so many ways that people identify—including (but not limited to) psychiatric survivor, mad, psychiatric service user, consumer, and mentally ill. I am looking for participants who identify with any, all, or none of these labels. While participants may have experience with psychiatric systems, it is not necessary to have such experience to participate. If you identify as LGBTQ and you feel like mental health has personally and directly affected you, I would like to hear from you.

Participants were recruited through posted notices in various health-related and queer-centred locations in both cities and through online means. Setting up interviews took place mainly over e-mail, with only a few interactions taking place over the telephone. Participants were given the option to choose any public space where they felt comfortable to do the interview. Participants were informed that the digitally recorded interview would be approximately 45–90 min in length, that they were free to withdraw from the study at any time without penalty, and that they were not required to answer any questions considered to be inappropriate, invasive, or offensive. All interviews were transcribed verbatim and anonymized. I performed multiple readings of each transcript to identify major themes related to the research using NVivo coding software.

Qualitative interviewing offered the opportunity to engage in meaningful dialogue and collect rich data. The participants were generous with their time and stories and shared their experiences extensively with me. The voices of mad LGBTQ people are rarely represented in textual sources, so my interviews are an invaluable source of first-person accounts of everyday life experience. Qualitative interviewing also allowed for flexibility in the interview process. I created an interview guide of open-ended questions about identity, health, work, and community that functioned as a base from which to start. Additional questions arose in the course of individual interviews. The open-ended interview format allowed me to follow up on comments made by participants with new questions, although I always returned to the interview guide in order to maintain some consistency among the interviews.

Another advantage of qualitative interviewing was that it allowed space for a more nuanced discussion of self-identity. As Warner (2004) points out, attempts to "quantify homosexuals, heterosexuals, etc., assumes a commonality between the individual's desires and lives that is suspect. Qualitative approaches have a better chance of accounting for queer experiences in the same terms as the actual people living these experiences" (p. 335). Warner is referring specifically to sexuality categories, but his point is also applicable to gender, race, class, and disability. Many of the participants engaged in complex discussions of their identities, which points to the difficulties of quantifying or simplifying any aspect of identity, not just sexual identity. For example, one participant described his race, class, sexuality, gender, and disability as "liminal" and "not easily defined as one or the other." He discussed being perceived as white, racialized, able-bodied, disabled, and a long list of queer, trans, and cisgender identities, depending on the circumstances. As he told me, "everything about me is so complicated and hard to point out." This participant's response highlights the limitations of identity categories and quantitative methods to capture the experiences of those who don't consistently pass as "one or the other." I found that qualitative interviewing allowed for more detailed discussions of these complexities. This was also true of discussions pertaining to identity, language, and mental health, or madness, which will be discussed in more detail in Chapter 3.

Demographics

The depth of discussion of identity elicited in the interviews was very important but also created challenges for my writing in terms of choosing language for referring to the study participants as a group. I asked participants to self-identify using whatever words they felt most comfortable with instead of choosing from a list of my creation. I made this choice because I believe that self-identification is particularly important for groups who have long been defined by others. When it came time to write a demographic account of the study participants, I struggled with creating a coherent description from the long and varied list of terms used by the participants, all of which did not easily lend itself to a chart. I made sense of this as follows.

The research participants were between the ages of 20 and 49, with 19 in their 20s, 13 in their 30s, and five in their 40s. In terms of gender, 18 participants identified as women and 14 identified as men. Of the women, five also identified as trans and/or genderqueer, as did seven of the men. The remaining five participants did not identify as men or women, instead using the term(s) trans and/or genderqueer. Many participants used more than one term to describe their sexuality: 23 identified as queer, eight as gay, five as lesbian, three as bisexual, two as pansexual or omnisexual, and one as heterosexual. It is important to note that the numbers for sexuality exceed the total number of participants (37) because many identified with more than one term. The participants also used many terms to describe their racial identifications, but broadly speaking 59% (22) of participants identified as white and 41% (15) identified as BIPOC. More specifically, two people identified as biracial or mixed race, four people identified as Métis, one person identified as Indigenous and Indonesian, one person identified as Black and Indigenous, three people identified as Black and of those three, two also identified as immigrants. One person identified as Middle Eastern and as an immigrant. One person identified as Brown and South Asian, one person identified as a person of colour and Korean, and one person identified as a person of colour and East Asian. Of the 22 people who identified as white, one also identified as Scottish, two as French Canadian, one as Portuguese, and one as South American. I did not specifically inquire about religion, but one white person identified as Jewish and one Middle Eastern person identified as Muslim. Just over half of the participants (19) identified as low income and the remaining 18 identified as middle class. In terms of disability, 19 participants identified as having one or more physical or mental disability.

Ethical Research Practice

A salient ethical issue specific to the people I interviewed was the prevalent, well-founded distrust of academic research and researchers based on the exploitation of marginalized groups by academics. Many scholars have pointed out that disabled people and specifically those with psychiatric disabilities have been subjected to unethical research practices and treated in ableist ways by researchers (see, for example, Oliver, 1992; Phillips, 2006; Shakespeare, 1996; Wilton, 2004). Research has often been used against the best interests of people with disabilities, and as Wilton (2004) argues, those working for psychiatric survivors' rights "have critically interrogated the motivations of researchers, and with good reason given the way in which scholarship has been used to legitimate the social and spatial exclusion of people with physical and psychiatric disabilities" (p. 117).

Many of the people I interviewed occupied multiple subject positions, which has often led to well-founded suspicion of academic research and researchers. Trans people, queer people, BIPOC, low income people, and people with disabilities have all been the object of knowledge production that has either erased their existence or otherwise exploited them. My population sample included people from all of these identity categories, many of whom, of course, identified with more than one. One way in which I tried to mitigate this was to offer a copy of the transcript of the interview to the participants in order for them to review it and make any changes before I made use of it. Twenty-six participants asked for a copy of the transcript and four made minor revisions by clarifying and adding additional comments.

It is important to note that what constitutes ethical research practice is subjective. As Phillips (2006) states, "the interpretation of what constitutes morally right and ethical research is a matter of agreement among members of a particular group at a given time; unsurprisingly, different groups will interpret this in different ways" (p. 175). The truth of this was highlighted during the research. One participant told me that upon hearing about her involvement in my study, a friend expressed dismay and concern that a researcher who was not professionally trained as a clinician would undertake research regarding mental health. This kind of concern is misguided and reflects an inability to conceptualize research about mental health outside of a medicalized context and positions mad people as fragile, volatile, and in need of professional medical protection.

This type of ethical concern when it comes to interviewing people about mental health is widespread. As Holland (2007) argues, ethics review boards often take a paternalistic approach when reviewing projects that propose to interview those who have been deemed mentally ill. Holland describes the ethics review feedback on her own proposed research regarding mental health, which questioned her qualifications as a humanities scholar and detailed concerns about her and her supervisory committee's lack of clinical training. The ethics board was also concerned about whether or not participants were "well enough" to participate in her project (Holland, 2007, p. 901). This concern raises questions about the definition of "well enough" and who gets to decide whether or not a participant qualifies as such. As Holland states, "the concept of 'well enough' is difficult to define and third-party judgments of 'well enough' potentially could be based on anything from perceiving people as too vulnerable, [to] too emotional, too angry, too resistant, too passive, or too much of a threat to the researcher" (p. 901).

Holland (2007) also points to the contested nature of mental illness and the failure of ethics boards to recognize this and understand mad people as those who have been medicalized rather than as patients (p. 900). She concludes that questioning the ability of those who have been deemed mentally ill to consent to participate in social research is in fact a violation of human rights and that ethics boards should not assume that ethical problems are present solely because of a medical diagnosis of mental illness (p. 910). Though I did not encounter the kinds of problems Holland describes during the ethics review process at York University where this study was approved, I believe that the aforementioned comments from a participant's friend reflect the attitudes Holland describes and draw attention to a significant issue in thinking through ethics in relation to my project.

This also highlights one of the contributions of my study: its approach from a Mad Studies perspective. The fact that I did not employ a positivist, medicalized approach was part of what enticed some interviewees to participate in my project. Many participants expressed a dislike for the paternalistic and pathologizing ways in which they had been treated by medical professionals. As a researcher coming from outside of medicine or psychology, I may have inspired more trust in some participants rather than less. For some participants, especially those who had experienced negative interactions with clinicians and medical professionals, my project was something they wanted to contribute to precisely because it offered ways of understanding mental health outside of a medicalized context.

Methods: Cultural Representations of Gender in Psychiatric Narratives (Study Two)

Chapter 5 draws on data from a second study, entitled Cultural Representations of Gender in Psychiatric Narratives. This project examined how psychiatry and the psychiatric institution are implicated in the organization of gender relations at the intersection of race, Indigeneity, sexuality, class, and disability. It sought to represent particular standpoints in an effort to investigate how psychiatric discourses participate in the (re)production and sanctioning of gendered ways of being distressed. In total, 161 psychiatric inpatient charts from a large psychiatric hospital in Ontario of patients discharged between January 2013 and September 2016 were examined. However, in this book I draw on a subsection of the larger dataset, focusing only on the charts of 16 trans and non-binary patients. For analyses of the larger dataset, I direct readers to the collection of essays titled *Interrogating Psychiatric Narratives of Distress: Documented Lives* (Daley & Pilling, 2021).

This study employed theories and methods informed by institutional ethnography (Smith, 2005), using interviews, observations, and texts as data to explore how experiences were bound up in social relations (Campbell & Gregor, 2004). Social relations refers to practices and activities that are coordinated and concerted by people's interactions with each other and with shared languages, taking "experience" beyond one's own motivations and intentions. Social relations include textually mediated practices in which texts have the power to "hold people to acting in particular ways" (Campbell & Gregor, 2004, p. 173). Institutional ethnography approaches challenge the idea that constructs, such as gender, race, sexuality, and class, can be abstracted from the practices of people acting within organizations and through texts. Instead, such constructs should be investigated as they emerge within a particular context and through people's activities (DeVault & McCoy, 2004). Using an institutional ethnography lens, the research team sought to reveal connections between the psychiatric inpatient charts, activities and texts that preceded them (e.g., organizational policies, everyday practices, dominant discourses on gender, race, sexuality, and class), and activities and texts that followed them (e.g., further charts, patient discharge notes, etc.). We considered the psychiatric chart as integral to human relations and lived experiences within the psychiatric institution, even when not all forms of data were available (as in the patient's own account of their experiences or exact transcripts of practitioner-patient interviews). Therefore, we viewed the psychiatric chart as both a product and a producer of people's activities with material, everyday implications.

Retrospective Chart Review

Charts belonging to people discharged between January 2013 and September 2016 were selected from anonymized discharge lists from four inpatient programs across the psychiatric institution. All charts were reviewed sequentially as they were listed on the discharge list until the target number of 30 charts from each unit was met. However, the initial extraction of 120 charts yielded only two charts belonging to trans people. I, therefore, performed a targeted extraction of 14 additional charts belonging to trans and non-binary people, as well as an additional 15 charts of lesbian, gay, bisexual, and queer people, and 12 charts belonging to bisexual people. A total of 161 charts were reviewed.

I reviewed all 161 charts in order to immerse myself in the data and manually transfer de-identified extracted data into individualized Word documents, which served as "texts" for analysis (Daley et al., 2012). Careful consideration was given to ensuring that data were not de-contextualized. For example, each excerpt was identified by the profession of the person documenting and the date of the inpatient admission during which the documentation occurred. Once these texts for analysis were created for every chart, the following steps were undertaken by two research team members (myself and Andrea Daley): (1) all the texts were read and a summary for each text was created, (2) each summary was read and a memo created for each summary to capture key themes across the texts, and (3) MP and AD read each other's memos with the intent to refine the key themes. Key themes were presented to the other three team members for feedback several times throughout this process. In this regard, critical discourse analysis was used to highlight the social and organizational categories of gender, sexuality, race, class, and disability that already existed in the charts and that functioned to shape chart documentation. Our readings explored ideological commitments underlying psychiatric charts including gendered, racialized, sexualized, and classed assumptions, meanings, and values (Lupton, 1992; Tupper, 2008).

Demographics

As described in more detail in Chapter 5, the institution's demographic data did not provide an accurate representation of patients' sexuality and gender due to the cisnormative practices used for gathering such data. Sexuality was often recorded inaccurately because gender identities were erroneously recorded as sexual orientation. Descriptions of patients' gender identities varied considerably across each chart, depending on the assessments of the practitioners who were documenting. It is important to note that the contradictions in demographic information suggest that while at times patients may have self-identified in a certain way to mental health practitioners, in many instances practitioners completed the form based on their own interpretation of the patient from their specific positionality. These documentation contradictions and silences speak to the violence inherent in quantifying identity in a drop-down format and institutional categorization practices that are neither neutral nor objective.

In order to provide a more respectful demographic description of the sample, I employed what I describe in Chapter 5 as a trans-positive lens; 1 sought to affirm trans and non-binary ways of being and resist the institution's imposition of cisnormative and transphobic understandings of gender. Based on my reading of the charts, I describe the demographics of the sample as follows. The 16 charts discussed in Chapter 5 include that of two Black, trans women, one Indigenous, trans woman, eight white, trans women/transfeminine people,[2] one white, trans man, and four white, non-binary people. In the case of four people, sexuality was erroneously recorded as transgender. For the remaining, one was recorded as bisexual, one as asexual, two as queer, five as unknown, two as heterosexual, and one was left blank. The patients ranged in age from 21 to 61, with a mean age of 33. Three people were employed, nine people were on social assistance, one person had no income, two people preferred not to answer, and one person's financial information was not recorded. Four of the 16 people had an income between $15,000 and $29,000, and the rest made below $15,000 or their income was not recorded. This places all of the people for whom financial information was recorded well below the poverty line in the city in which they lived. For a more fulsome description of the methodology for this project, including a discussion of limitations and research ethics, see Daley and Pilling (2021). This study received ethics approval from the psychiatric institution from which the charts were reviewed and from all participating universities.

Acknowledgements Sections of this appendix draw on an earlier publication by the author: Daley, A., & Pilling, M. D. (2021). Introduction: Psychiatric documentation, power, and violence. In A. Daley & M. D. Pilling (Eds.), *Interrogating psychiatric narratives of madness: Documented lives* (pp. 1–31). Palgrave Macmillan.

Notes

1. For a discussion of participants' workplace experiences, see Pilling (2013).
2. Given the lack of information about self-identification, I use the more expansive term "transfeminine" in cases where it was unclear if the person would have identified as a trans woman. I use transfeminine as an umbrella term to capture all those who identified on a feminine gender spectrum in contrast to their sex/gender assigned at birth but who may or may not have identified as a trans woman. In doing so, I recognize that the terms "transfeminine" and "transmasculine" can be seen as replicating a binary view of gender.

References

Campbell, M., & Gregor, F. (2004). Theory "in" everyday life. In W. K. Carroll (Ed.), *Critical strategies for social research* (pp. 170–180). Canadian Scholars Press.

Daley, A., Costa, L., & Ross, L. (2012). (W)righting women: Constructions of gender, sexuality and disorder through psychiatric documentation practices. *Culture, Health and Sexuality, 14*(8), 955–969. https://doi.org/10.1080/13691058.2012.712718

Daley, A., & Pilling, M. D. (2021). *Interrogating psychiatric narratives of madness: Documented lives*. Palgrave Macmillan.

DeVault, M. L., & McCoy, L. (2004). Institutional ethnography: Using interviews to investigate ruling relations. In W. K. Carroll (Ed.), *Critical strategies for social research* (pp. 191–205). Canadian Scholars Press.

Holland, K. (2007). The epistemological bias of ethics review. *Qualitative Inquiry, 13*(6), 895–913. https://doi.org/10.1177/1077800407304469

Lupton, D. (1992). Discourse analysis: A new methodology for understanding the ideologies of health and illness. *Australian Journal of Public Health, 16*(2), 145–150. https://doi.org/10.1111/j.1753-6405.1992.tb00043.x

Oliver, M. (1992). Changing the social relations of research production? *Disability, Handicap & Society, 7*(2), 101–114. https://doi.org/10.1080/02674649266780141

Phillips, R. (2006). Consumer participation in mental health research. *Social Policy Journal of New Zealand, 27*, 171–182. Retrieved August 19, 2021, from https://www.msd.govt.nz/documents/about-msd-and-our-work/publications-resources/journals-and-magazines/social-policy-journal/spj27/27-pages171-182.pdf

Pilling, M. D. (2013). Invisible identity in the workplace: Intersectional madness and processes of disclosure at work. *Disability Studies Quarterly, 33*(1). https://dsq-sds.org/article/view/3424/3204

Shakespeare, T. (1996). Rules of engagement: Doing disability research. *Disability and Society, 11*, 115–120. https://doi.org/10.1080/09687599650023380

Smith, D. E. (2005). *Institutional ethnography: A sociology for people.* AltaMira Press.

Statistics Canada. (2013a, May 9). *2011 National household survey: Immigration, citizenship, place of birth, ethnicity, visible minorities, religion and Aboriginal peoples: Backgrounder.* Retrieved August 25, 2021, from https://www.toronto.ca/wp-content/uploads/2017/10/9793-2011-NHS-Backgrounder-Immigration-Citizenship-Place-of-Birth-Ethnicity-Visible-Minorities-Religion-and-Aboriginal-Peoples-.pdf

Statistics Canada. (2013b, September 11). *Winnipeg, CY, Manitoba (Code 4611040) (table). National Household Survey (NHS) Profile. 2011 National Household Survey. Statistics Canada Catalogue no. 99-004-XWE.* Ottawa. Retrieved August 25, 2021, from https://www12.statcan.gc.ca/nhs-enm/2011/dp-pd/prof/details/page.cfm?Lang=E&Geo1=CSD&Code1=4611040&Data=Count&SearchText=Winnipeg&SearchType=Begins&SearchPR=01&TABID=1&A1=All&B1=All&Custom=

Tupper, K. W. (2008). Drugs, discourses and education: A critical discourse analysis of a high school drug education text. *Discourse: Studies in the Cultural Politics of Education, 29*(2), 223–238. https://doi.org/10.1080/01596300801966864

Warner, D. N. (2004). Towards a queer research methodology. *Qualitative Research in Psychology, 4*(1), 321–337. https://doi.org/10.1191/147808870 4qp021oa

Wilton, R. D. (2004). Keeping your distance: Balancing political engagement and scientific autonomy with a psychiatric consumer/survivor group. In D. Fuller & R. Kitchin (Eds.), *Radical geography/critical praxis: Making a difference beyond the academy* (pp. 116–131). Praxis (e)Press.

Index

www.ingramcontent.com/pod-product-compliance
Ingram Content Group UK Ltd.
Pitfield, Milton Keynes, MK11 3LW, UK
UKHW020113140425
457327UK00002B/2